No Life Too Small

Love and loss at the world's first animal hospice

ALEXIS FLEMING

QUERCUS

First published in hard back in Great Britain in 2021 by Quercus Editions Ltd

This paperback edition published in 2022 by

QUERCUS

Quercus Editions Ltd
Carmelite House
50 Victoria Embankment
London EC4Y 0DZ

An Hachette UK company

A CIP catalogue record for this book is available
from the British Library

PB ISBN 978 1 52941 167 6
Ebook ISBN 978 1 52941 165 2

10 9 8 7 6 5 4 3 2 1

Typeset by CC Book Production
Printed and bound in Great Britain by Clays Ltd, Elcograf S.p.A.

Papers used by Quercus Editions are from well-managed forests and other responsible sources.

Alexis Fleming, 38, grew up in Kilmarnock and studied geography at Strathclyde University. She has worked as an animal rights campaigner and in 2013 she started a charity called Pounds for Poundies to help rescue unclaimed dogs from being put down which raised £10K in its first week. She's a committed vegan and, as well as the hospice, she also runs the Karass Sanctuary where she cares for neglected and terminally ill farm animals, many of which have been saved from the slaughterhouse.

Alexis's story has been covered by ITV, the BBC and has featured in the *Sun* and the *Guardian*. A short documentary called *Crannog* about the hospice premiered at the Edinburgh International Film Festival and has been shown around the world. It was recently shortlisted for 'outstanding non-fiction short film' and is up for an award in New York this month (February 2020).

In 2020 Alexis was featured in BBC Three's 'Amazing Humans' series and a clip of her went viral.

For Maggie, who took and left the biggest pieces.

CONTENTS

See **www.nolifetoosmall.co.uk**
for accompanying pictures and extra stories
for each chapter.

CHAPTER ONE

'Maggie, d'ye think yer funny?'

Aye, you're going to have a lot of explaining to do when you get home . . .

I was standing in a car park in a part of York that I didn't know. I fidgeted with the notes in the pocket of my coat, my palms sweaty and cold. Christmas music and hot air seeped out of the automatic doors from the warmth of the supermarket. The midwinter darkness wrapped around me, as heavy as my growing dread.

I called again; straight to voicemail. I tried again. And again.

I looked around at the unfamiliar housing estate. How long should I wait? How many times do I call? When do I give up?

It was starting to dawn on me that I might be too late. I should have left work and come sooner, offered more money, worried more. I checked the time on my phone: 16.34. One more try.

Glancing up from my phone, I tensed; passing under the glow of the street lights, a man was coming towards me. He was a wiry guy in his thirties, walking quickly, eyes down, looking at his phone. In the orange gloom, it took a moment for my eyes and brain to make sense of what I was seeing. But it was . . . it was her! The skinny bullmastiff trotting behind him had no collar and no lead, but she followed him obediently along the pavement, trailing his ankles. They walked over to me, the dog cowering nervously behind him. It was clear that she was terrified of him.

'You here for the dog?' he asked, glancing up from his phone. I nodded nervously, my mouth dry.

'Got the cash?'

'Aye. A hundred quid. I thought maybe you'd given her to the other guy.'

'What? Oh, no, he didn't turn up. Do you still want it?'

'Aye. Here . . .'

I held out the money. He gave it a quick check and pocketed it. I opened the hatch of my battered old Mazda and signalled for her to jump in. 'Come on, darling,' I urged her gently, patting the duvet in the open boot.

She looked up at me with huge, fearful brown eyes, but didn't budge. *Come on, darling, get in.* I wanted this to be over.

'You heard her. Get in.'

With his boot, he shoved her towards the car. She flinched and instinctively did as she was told, and I quickly brought the door down. Comforting words would come later; right now, my only task was to get her safe.

'Right, cheers,' he said, and, without a goodbye or a backward glance to the dog, he walked off. I could be anyone, out to do anything to her, but he'd got his cash. I watched him leave, his eyes back on his phone, the skinny, terrified dog who had loyally followed him and obeyed his every word already forgotten as he turned the corner into the darkness.

I looked up and exhaled with relief. *Thank you.*

Opening the boot of the car was too risky, so I climbed into the back seat. I had to be careful around any new dog, especially one who was clearly so confused and afraid. I didn't know much about bullmastiffs, though I remembered reading that they are very loyal and sometimes wary of strangers. But, looking at this poor, frightened dog huddled in my boot, I wasn't alarmed.

'Hi, darling.' I held out my hand for her to sniff. 'You're a nice lass, aren't you? Try not to be scared.' She stared back at me, her eyes wide, confused and anxious. Unsure, she gave my hand a quick, tentative sniff.

'It's going to be OK, I promise. Let's get you home.'

It was rush hour in York's nightmare of a road network, and the journey took forever, but she didn't move or make a sound throughout. Crawling along the gridlocked road, I glanced in the rear-view mirror. I could see her silhouetted, sitting bolt upright, her floppy ears bouncing in rhythm with our stops and starts. Even when I stopped to buy food for my unexpected guest, I got back in the car to find her in exactly the same position. Her lack of reaction worried me, but I was also quite glad of the silence, as it gave me time to think.

I turned into the car park at the block of flats where I lived and pulled into the bay marked with my flat number. I turned the key in the ignition and shifted round in my seat to look behind me at the dark outline in the back, the unknown entity I'd invited into my life on a momentary whim. I could feel her looking back at me through the darkness. Turning around, I closed my eyes and let my head fall forward. *Bloody hell.* The adrenaline was fading, and reality was dawning.

When I'd left home this morning, it hadn't been my intention to come back nine hours later with a dog. My husband Chris and I were renting an apartment where we weren't allowed pets. I worked packing boxes in the warehouse of an optical components company, and this morning had been the same as any other. As usual, I was first in, and I'd got the heaters fired up and put the radio and the kettle on. It took me a while to get going in the morning; I was always tired, as tired when I woke up as when I went to bed, and I was finding it harder to explain away the unusual aches, pains and weariness that were starting to noticeably slow me down. It was mid-December and it was going to be a busy day as we rushed to get orders out before the Christmas break, and I was tired just thinking about it. I'd sat down at the computer with a cup of tea to help get me going and started to check emails and orders.

I'd never been a big fan of Christmas, and I was feeling particularly disheartened and cynical about it this year. Bombarded by adverts, tinsel and forced merriment that disguised the darker reality lurking behind the glossily marketed festivities – debt, stress, loneliness, old dogs dumped to make way for new puppies – I really wasn't in the mood for it. I felt empty and restless.

Growing up as an only child, my best friend and playmate was Trouvee, a Staffordshire bull terrier cross, whom my mum and dad had found as a skinny, neglected, traumatised pup, dumped close to a bridge in Glasgow city centre, in the 1970s. She'd hated kids until I was born, and then she had a total change of heart and decided I was her baby, her wean, and she'd have protected me with her life. I was twelve when Trouvee died, and in her memory, my mum, Flora, started a cat rescue, which she ran from our house. The scale of the stray-cat problem meant it quickly took over our home and our lives. I once came home after a five-hour shift working at the local cinema to find seventeen kittens in my bedroom.

'Where – how – did you find seventeen kittens in the last five hours, Mum? Four, aye! Five at a push, that's not unheard of. But seventeen?! Any chance they're going to stop playing chases over me while I'm trying to sleep? And anything you can do about them thinking I'm a luxury heated litter tray you've installed for them? One of them's peed on my pillow, Mum!'

She came back a few minutes later and handed me a plastic tarpaulin to sleep under. Problem solved.

I was used to the highs and lows and the willing sacrifices needed to share home and life with society's furry waifs and strays, but sadly I'd never been settled enough to have an animal pal of my own. Chris and I had met when we'd both worked at the Odeon cinema in Kilmarnock. I was nineteen and it was a student job while I did my degree; he was a year older than me and had just graduated. We went travelling together when I was twenty-one, including a year living in Australia, where I worked as a campaigner for an animal-welfare charity. While I was there, I was delighted to discover Edgar's Mission, a sanctuary for rescued farm animals near Melbourne, and, from the second I met Pam, who ran it, that was my weekends and days off sorted. I just loved those days cleaning out chicken coops and pigsties, and babysitting piglets and cockerels. I was in my element. Back home, Chris and I got married, but hadn't ever settled in one place. Chris worked in the hotel industry, so we moved around a lot, and his latest job had landed us here in York.

I had friends who ran rescues, and, since getting back, I'd taken in dogs and fostered them for a few weeks until they found a new home, but I'd never been in a position to keep any of them permanently.

I still wasn't.

But, this morning, without thinking about it enough to dissuade myself, I'd clicked onto an online ad site. As always, there were pages and pages of unwanted dogs for sale, alongside the worn-out excuses that always accompanied them. Scrolling down, a photograph caught my attention: a forlorn-looking brindle bullmastiff sitting on a wicker chair, discarded kids' toys and other rubbish strewn in the garden around her. She was small and skinny, and she looked hauntingly sad.

I read the advert twice, hoping that I'd misunderstood it the first time:

Bought this bitch for breeding. Had twelve puppies but ten died so it's no use to me. At my girlfriend's house but she doesn't want it and she's beating it up. 10 months old. £100.

It.

She was far too young to have puppies; she wasn't much more than a puppy herself. I reread the words, and the decision made itself. My mouth was dry and adrenaline had started to flow and do its thing. Heart in charge and head struggling to keep up, I picked up the phone and dialled the number.

A disinterested voice answered. 'The dog? Oh, right, yeah. Some bloke's already offered me a gold signet ring and a motorcycle helmet. I'd rather have cash, but it needs to go,' he told me, 'and he can collect it this morning.'

A gold signet ring and a motorcycle helmet? What the hell? Within seconds, I was invested in this dog I'd never met, and I was determined to get her away from this guy, and the bloke who wanted to swap her for a ring and a helmet. I had to give him a reason to wait, and guessed that persuading him I was going to give her a wonderful home wasn't going to be what did it. Steadying the wobble in my voice, I gave it my best shot: 'I can't get there until after work, but I'll give you the full amount, a hundred pounds cash. That's worth more than what the other guy offered. I can be there just after four. Tell me where to meet you.'

The promise of cash over a motorcycle helmet had swayed him. Quarter past four, the Co-op car park, in a dodgy part of the city I'd never been to before.

Now, here I was, down a hundred pounds, up a bullmastiff, and with no plan as to how I was going to wedge her into my not-at-all-bullmastiff-compatible life. I briefly toyed with the idea of regretting it all, but I was in it now and the dog-shaped shadow behind me told me I'd done the right thing.

Anxious, I knew I needed to break the news to Chris, who was upstairs in our flat, unaware of my latest escapade. I was ashamed and felt really guilty, but I hadn't told him beforehand because I didn't want to be talked out of it. I got my phone out of my pocket.

'A dog? Alexis . . . how? Where? You've only been at work! And we're not allowed pets.'

'I know. I'm sorry. I saw her online.'

'She can't stay. This is ridiculous. You should have asked me first.'

'Look, I'm sorry, I really am. I saw her and I had to help her, Chris. He was going to swap her for a motorcycle helmet! His girlfriend was beating her up. I know I should have asked you. I'm sorry. But, once I knew about her, I had to do something. I'm sorry, I really am . . .' I was rambling. I knew I was in the wrong, here, and I should have told him.

'What are you going to do with her?'

'I don't know,' I said quietly, my voice deflating along with my previous certainty.

He was pretty upset with me. Chris cared, but we didn't see things the same way. It *was* a selfish move – I'd taken on a dog without thinking about the impact it would have on Chris – and it was going to cause a lot of hassle with our landlord. Aye, it was fair enough. I'd have been upset at me, too.

A few minutes later, Chris came down to the car park.

'Alexis . . .' He opened the back door of the car and looked at me.

I was crouching on the back seat, reaching into the boot to stroke the huge, brown, sad, smelly, unknown dog. Ashamed, thrilled, relieved, worried, certain and uncertain, I looked back at Chris.

'What's she called?' he asked.

It hadn't even occurred to me. 'I don't know; I didn't ask. Maggie? Aye, why not? Maggie. She's called Maggie.'

I was starting to panic and regret it all, but I had no choice, now; I'd got myself into this and I had to keep going. I took a deep breath. 'Right, Maggie, shall we get you upstairs?'

I didn't know her, and she was in a very confusing and scary situation. She might bolt, or fear might get the better of her and she might decide to get an attack in first. Carefully, I opened the boot and we looked at each other for a few moments. I got an overwhelming feeling that she had no intention of going anywhere or of hurting me. Relieved, I fastened a collar around her neck and attached a lead.

'Do you need a wee, sweetheart?'

Chris had gone ahead of us, and he stood at the top of the two flights of stairs, holding the door open for Maggie and me.

'She seems scared,' he said. 'What's her story?'

I explained.

'What are you going to do? She can't stay here.'

'Aye, I know, I know . . .' I still didn't have a plan. 'I'm not sure, yet. But I'll work something out,' I told him, and myself.

We walked through the front door and along the hall to the open-plan living room and kitchen. Now, in the light of the flat, I could see the bags of exhaustion under Maggie's eyes.

'Right, darling, let's get you settled . . .' She was confused, but resigned to what was happening. I guess it was just another move in her chaotic life, and she'd learned that there was nothing good to come of making a fuss. I unclipped her lead and reached past her head to pick up the bag of shopping. Her belly hit the floor, flat as she could make herself.

Suddenly, I remembered the words of the online ad: *she's beating it up*. Until an hour ago, that had been her reality. Beatings, puppies, hunger, fear.

'Oh, darling, it's OK. No one's going to hurt you now.' I tried to reassure her, but she had no reason to believe me.

I sat down on the floor next to her, both of us leaning against the sofa, and started gently stroking the top of her head. It was the first time I'd noticed how dirty and dull her fur was. She had a beautiful brindle coat – dark brown, flecked with oranges and golds – and she had a long wavy white bib, running up under her chin and down her chest. I felt her tense at my touch as I slowly put my arm over her, and, as I gently ran my hand over her back, flecks of dandruff fell to the floor. I'd noticed earlier that her teats were sagging, full of the milk for her puppies who had died. They didn't look good, and there was a chance they were infected.

'Do you mind if I just reach under here, darlin' . . . ?' I already felt that Maggie was a gentle soul. But if she was infected and sore, and not used to kind hands, she might not react well to me touching her painful, swollen belly. She watched my hand wearily as I reached round. Her teats were hot and her whole belly was covered in open, seeping, crusty sores that looked like terrible acne.

'Bloody hell, what's this? Chris, look at her belly. She's covered in scabs, and she's all infected.'

We stood together, looking at her slumped on her side, exhausted, worried, one paw raised, ready for us to do whatever we wanted to her.

'She must be in a lot of pain.' Chris winced. It was difficult to look at.

'Aye, I need to get her to the vet tomorrow. But before anything else, she needs a good feed and a good night's sleep.'

I improvised and filled two pasta bowls – one with food, and the other with water. She was ravenous, but fear and worry had a good grip on her. I backed away to give her some space, and it wasn't long before hunger and temptation edged her cautiously towards the food, and she took a few hesitant mouthfuls. Soon the food bowl was empty and drools of water hung from her jowls. She shook her head, and a stray strand of saliva hit the fridge and started to gloop down the door.

'We better get that before Chris sees it, Maggie! Nae drool on the walls, OK?' Which reminded me: I had to ring our landlord and confess that I'd suddenly acquired a dog, who was now busy furnishing our no-pets-allowed flat with strings of dog-foody saliva.

Later that evening, as Maggie was cautiously sniffing her way along the grass verge outside our block of flats, I finally pestered myself into biting the bullet and calling our landlord.

'She was being mistreated,' I explained. 'It's only temporary – just for a few days, until Christmas Eve, until I find her a space in kennels. I'm going to see if I can take her to work with me, and I'll make sure she doesn't cause any bother or do any damage. I'm sorry to have to ask, I just had to do something.' I waited nervously for his reaction.

'Thanks for being honest with me,' he said. 'And thanks for helping her. I've got a dog myself. He's fast asleep in front of the fire, just now – all dogs deserve that. Please try and make sure she doesn't cause any damage or upset the neighbours, and good luck finding her a great new home.'

What a relief.

That was one hurdle crossed. I'd call my boss in the morning and ask if it was OK to take Maggie in with me for the next couple of days, until we closed for Christmas break. She seemed like a quiet dog, and I just had to hope she didn't have a hidden penchant for office destruction.

Home from our walk, Maggie and I sat next to each other on the living-room floor, warming up. She wasn't even a year old and already life was taking its toll on her body. I took another look at her swollen, red, scabby belly. Growing, feeding and caring for her pups – and, I guessed, a bad diet and not much concern about a few missed mealtimes – had left her skinny and malnourished. If it had ever been an option, relaxation had been out of the question for so long that it wasn't going to come easy to her, but she looked utterly exhausted. 'You've really been through it, haven't you? Come on, Maggie, it's been quite a day. Let's get to bed.'

Chris was already asleep when Maggie and I went through to the bedroom. 'Come, lie down, darling. This should be comfy for you.' I watched her from the bathroom as I brushed my teeth, sniffing the blankets I'd laid out for her next to my side of the bed, starting to build a picture of her new world. She pawed at them a few times, turned around and lay down.

Trying not to disturb her, I manoeuvred over the pile of blankets and got into bed. Lying there in the dark, I took a few deep breaths and tried to make sense of things and get my thoughts in order. What a day it had been!

I was weary, but I was ready for and expecting an unsettled night. Maggie's life and world had changed completely in the last few hours, into something unrecognisable, and first nights in strange places are often difficult at the best of times. She was exhausted, though, and I hoped that would override her fear and she'd get the rest she needed. I needn't have worried. A few minutes was all it took for our breathing to slow and for two overwhelmed bodies to fall asleep next to each other.

Aside from a couple of wee puddles and Maggie's dinner making a reappearance on the carpet, we both slept well. Nerves and anxiety do funny things to our insides.

While we were on our early-morning walk, I called my boss. 'So, John, there's this dog . . .'

He knew me well enough to not be remotely surprised, and his cheerful Labrador, Jake, was already the office morale booster, so the proposition of a dog in the office wasn't out of the question. He was happy for Maggie to come into the warehouse for a couple of days before we closed for the Christmas break. I was grateful for his kindness and understanding – and very relieved, because I didn't have another plan.

Another hurdle cleared. Keep going . . .

It had only been twenty-four hours since we met, but Maggie and I were getting into the swing of things. We began to develop a routine, our friendship growing with every jaunt down the stairs for a sniff and a wee, and every moment spent cuddling on the living-room floor. There were a few accidents at work and at home, but nothing that a bottle of antibac spray and a few rolls of kitchen towel couldn't rectify. At work, she lay on her duvet under the packing bench where I spent my days, contentedly entertaining herself with a large chew toy and quickly making pals with the folk in the office. She was eating well, and antibiotics and some pain relief from the vet were getting to work on the discomfort of the infection that raged through her body. It was easy – much easier than I'd anticipated. We fitted together, somehow.

That weekend, we went for our first proper walk along an old railway embankment nearby. I wasn't ready to test Maggie's off-lead skills just yet, so she stayed attached to me by a longish lead. It was a bright winter day and the sun hung low in the sky, blinding me as a mother and daughter stopped to chat.

'We saw her coming – she's beautiful!' Smiling, they bent down to speak to Maggie. 'What's her name? I know it sounds silly, but when we saw her, we both said that she seems like a really gentle soul, and we had to stop and meet her. I hope you don't mind.'

Pride warmed my chest as I told them her story. Maggie's life had been chaos, fear, worry, and she'd never known kindness or had a friend. She had no reason to trust any of us. But she did. In the last few days, I'd watched as she welcomed new people like old friends, quietly and gently, giving them a paw if they asked and gently returning the kisses folk gave her. Her eyes had softened and a few good nights' sleep had taken care of the bags under them, while good, regular food and medication to treat her ills had given her a spring in her step. She was coming alive.

Mags and I were growing closer and more relaxed and confident with each other with every walk, car trip and cuddle on the couch, but we still had a long way to go. Her life of dodging angry hands or feet, missed meals, being passed from pillar to post and desperately trying to protect her pups in the midst of it all had made Maggie used to living on her nerves. Sometimes, when I made a sudden move or turned around too quickly in the kitchen, she'd plaster herself to the opposite wall, ears back, eyes huge, head down, making herself as small a target as she could. Old memories and habits die hard, especially ones we've developed to protect ourselves. Love and time needed to work their magic.

Christmas had come round fast, and so had another hurdle. Chris and I were going to a wedding in the Highlands between Christmas and New Year, and kennels would be booked up over the holidays. Where was Maggie going to go? Stuck, I did what any self-respecting daughter would do and called my mum and dad. Happy to help – and unsurprised – my dad, Archie, agreed to look after Maggie for a couple of days.

The wedding was wedding-y, and although I passed the time chatting to folk and even let myself be coaxed into a couple of dances, I couldn't stop thinking about Maggie, and about how tired I was. It was only a few days until she was due to go to stay at my friend Heather's boarding kennels, where she was going to be spayed, chipped and vaccinated, and then they would find her a fantastic new home. Heather was very careful and I trusted that she would only let Maggie go to live with people who would love and be kind to her. I had no doubt that she'd find a home where Maggie would be really happy and live a wonderful life.

Head down, embarrassed, I ran to the toilets. Alone in a cubicle, I was grateful for the music, laughter and clinking glasses that masked my sobs. I realised I didn't want Maggie to be loved by someone else. She already had a person who loved her. Me. I loved her.

I dabbed my eyes with cold water and waited until the redness had calmed down. Back in the festivities, I didn't need to make up an excuse to return to the chalet early; the familiar and overwhelming exhaustion had taken hold, along with the almost unbearable pain that always started after I ate and sapped me of all my energy and enthusiasm. For me, leaving a get-together early was becoming the norm.

Far enough away from the party, in the woods that surrounded the hotel, it was blissfully quiet, dark and calm in the chalet. I lay half-dressed in bed, teeth unbrushed, face unwashed, and cried. I barely had the energy to keep my eyes open, but, as usual, my mind was in overdrive. An hour later, I'd thought about it enough.

I inhaled and let out a long breath. I'd made up my mind. I loved Maggie, and she and I were staying together. Smiling, thrilled, I rang Dad.

'She's been wandering around the house looking for you,' he told me.

I smiled.

'I took her for a walk round the woods, today. I tried to take her across the stream, but she didn't know what water was.'

'I'm not going to give her up, Dad. She's staying with me.'

It wasn't going to be easy, but I was determined. I turned over to go to sleep, thinking about the exciting new future that had just appeared in front of me.

'Chris, I want to keep Maggie.' It was the morning after the wedding, and I tried to keep my voice low as the other people staying in the chalet with us got ready for breakfast.

'Alexis, you know we can't have dogs in the flat. You can't keep her.' Exasperated, his voice grew louder.

'Just listen to me, please. Our lease is up in eight weeks. I'll find us somewhere else to live, somewhere that allows dogs. I know you like the flat, I do too, but I'll look at houses near my work so I can go home to see her at lunchtime. I've called Heather and arranged that she can stay with her until I find somewhere. She's staying with us, Chris. I can't . . . I don't want to be without her.'

He closed his eyes and sighed, and my heart tightened.

*

17

NO LIFE TOO SMALL

I spent the first few weeks of January house hunting and calling Heather every few days for an update.

'She loves a run around with the other dogs. She's such a nice lassie, she gets on with everyone.' Heather was getting really fond of Mags.

'She is, isn't she? Right, are you sitting down? I found a house for us! We get the keys on 19 February. Is it OK for Dad to come and pick her up on his way down to help us move?'

Our new home was a semi with a garden in the suburbs of York. It was close to where I worked, so I would be able to go home at lunchtime to let Mags out for a wee.

The day before Maggie was due to arrive, I saw a post on Facebook about a blind husky called Jack who was going to be killed the next day because his people were having an unexpected baby. *Poor guy . . . Ach, well, two dogs are as easy as one dog.*

Jack arrived an hour before Maggie, and after he managed to lock himself in the bathroom and destroy the bath, dig a hole in the door and eat through the U-bend, I realised that, when one of those dogs was a half-bonkers, howling, spinning, blind husky who eats toilets, it was absolutely *not* easier to have two dogs. It was always my plan to find him a new home, but funnily enough, there wasn't a queue forming round the block. Jack and I had a strained relationship; he hated sneezing, and he made me sneeze. When I went into a room, he left. He'd sleep on my bed all day, and then go downstairs so he didn't have to listen to me sneeze all night. We muddled through, though, and, although it took a long time, eventually Jack found his way to Matt. Matt already had a couple of huskies and a job that took him into the forests in Cumbria every day, where Jack would be able to go with him. It was love at first sight when they met, and the ungrateful wee sod was curled up asleep on Matt's knee within half an hour.

Mags and I carried on where we left off, delighted to be reunited. I was tired and sore, and by the time I got home from work, I was usually pretty done in, so we spent our evenings lying on the couch, under a blanket, dozing, while Chris watched TV. During the week, we walked around the wee pond in the estate where we lived, and on weekends, we made an afternoon of it and went to the local country park for our walks. Every few weeks, we went up to see Mum and Dad in Kilmarnock, and Maggie had become part of the furniture there, too. But we were always happiest when we were hanging out at home together.

'Come on, Mags,' I said, heaving myself out from under the blanket on the couch. 'Time for night-night wees.'

It wasn't that late, but I was fading and I needed my bed.

'Maggie . . . come on, rouse yourself!'

Nothing.

'Maggie! I know yer no' sleeping, I can see you opening one eye. Up, out of bed!'

Nothing.

'Maggie, d'ye think yer funny?'

Thud. An involuntary wag.

'Got ye! I knew you were pretending. Out for a wee.'

She sighed, stretched and walked to the back door, her tail wagging in anticipation of her last few sniffs of the day, before toast and bed.

CHAPTER TWO

Futures

Raring to go, Maggie bounced into the car. 'Where to, Mags? Loch Morlich? Our Rothie walk? Nah, Loch Morlich. It might be nice enough for a wee paddle, today.' As I closed the boot, different types of pain went up, down and through me. Knowing the script, I steadied myself as I limped round the car and eased myself into the driver's seat. 'It's gaunnie be a slow one today, Mags.'

Chris's job in the hotel industry had relocated us again, and home was now a rented bungalow just outside Aviemore, in the far north of Scotland. I was grateful to be back in Scotland, and especially grateful to be living where we did. It wasn't any further from my family and friends than York had been, and because Mum, Dad and I used to come to the area for holidays in our caravan, it was familiar and welcoming. As a toddler, I'd spent my summers exploring the hills with Dad and Trouvee, filling Mum's pockets with pine cones and telling stories about fairies, and I'd amused myself for hours in the wee stream that ran alongside the campsite, its never-ending possibilities satisfying the never-ending imagination of a solitary, insomniac toddler.

We turned on to the ski road, heading towards the mountains. I glanced at Mags in the rear-view mirror, tongue lolling and ears bouncing, and wished she could give me some of her enthusiasm and energy. A sign at the side of the road told me that there was danger of forest fires. *Aw, is there, aye? It hasnae stopped raining for weeks . . . More bloody danger of the sign floating away.*

The familiar waymarkers held their positions along the road – lay-by on the right, the gnarly bones of a long-dead tree on the left. The ski road takes winter and summer tourists from Aviemore up to the walks and slopes of the Cairngorm Mountain, dividing a few clusters of houses and a pine forest, dropping people off at lochs and campsites along the way. It climbs and hairpins its way up the mountain and, above the treeline, delivers awesome views of the distant hills, deep lochs and toy cars crawling along the roads through the intriguing, haunting space of the national park below.

On the next corner, we passed the crumpled road sign – a mess of metal, using a tree to hold itself up – a permanent reminder of someone's really bad day. The roads around Aviemore are scenic, but they are also notorious; speed, brutal winters, momentary lapses of concentration, tragic encounters between car and deer, and plain rotten luck on a sharp bend are the main contributors to many bad, sometimes really bad, accidents. A dark thought flickered through my mind. *What would it be like to just lose control . . . ?*

A spasm grabbed a handful of my intestines and started twisting and clawing, my body instinctively clenching and doubling me over. Gritting my teeth and steadying my breath, I tried to stay focused on the road ahead. The spasm eased into a temporary lull and the nausea started to rise. Seconds later, another spasm above my right hip began swelling to its crescendo. I gripped the steering wheel and groaned. *Please, just for a while, let it stop.*

Constant pain and crippling fatigue had come to make every moment a test of endurance, an unending cycle of limping across the finishing line of one marathon and stumbling straight into another. A desolate numbness had slicked across my mind, leeching the life from everything it touched. I felt like I was grasping on to something steep and slippery in the dark, terrified of what I was holding on to, and terrified of the pit I'd fall into if I let go.

I glanced back at Maggie, cheerful and ready for our walk. Straight ahead, the wide-trunked pine, my old friend, rose from the grass verge, dependably solid and immovable. The road veered around it, insisting that I did, too. *What if I didn't want to go around it? What then?*

Anticipation getting the better of her, Maggie shifted in the boot. Another shock of pain rippled out from my guts. Weary, I glanced into the rear-view mirror. An excited face was looking back at me, eager for her paddle in the loch. I could hardly think how I was going to make it to the car park, never mind drag myself round the loch. 'You looking forward to it, Mags? Not far, now. We're almost there . . .' I took a deep breath, and obligingly followed the path of the road around the tree and on towards the loch. *Fucking coward . . .*

In our new home, living among the mountains, lochs, pine forests and remote, desolate beauty of the Cairngorms National Park, Maggie and I were spoiled for walks: woodland walks, sniff walks, paddling walks, sandy beach walks. In the off season, most days we wouldn't see anyone else; it was just the two of us, and miles of pine-needled paths and trees in all directions. On good days, when mind and body allowed, I loved our walks. I'd watch Mags splashing and let my thoughts wander as I threw stones and sticks into the turquoise shallows of *An Lochan Uaine*, the Green Loch, shaking my head and laughing as she tried to get a stick that was just . . . out . . . of . . . reach, gripping on to the sandy bed with her toenails. 'There's not much point in shaking yerself dry while yer still *in* the water, Mags!'

In the summer, when the beaches and paths were busy with families enjoying themselves, she'd confidently pad along, wagging her tail, and casually wander over to introduce herself to everyone who looked her way. She loved meeting new dogs, and quite often she'd meet one as daft as her and they'd run in circles for a while, taunt each other with their favourite sticks and share some good sniffs. To Mags, everyone was a friend. She'd nuzzle into strangers, looking up at them, doe-eyed, tongue hanging out, relishing the attention. On more than one occasion, up at Loch Morlich, she followed her nose to a family picnic; realising what was happening too late, I arrived out of breath and apologising as she cheerfully explored the spread. Somehow, she almost always managed to trot away with a reward for her cheek.

Out in the woods and the comforting aloneness, I talked to her, talked to myself, some days buoyed and propelled by thoughts, other days crumpled to the ground by them. Sometimes I cried and sometimes I blethered to Mum on the phone, and there were days when any sense of purpose was a distant memory, and I just put one foot in front of the other, not really caring much where the steps took me. On days when we had a bit of a spring in our step, we walked further, up past the Rothie campsite and towards the Lairig Ghru, the pass that cut through the mountains, and the Chalamain Gap, a boulder field where Dad and I had walked throughout my childhood and into my early twenties. Nothing was as thrilling as finding a path across boulders the size of small cars, one slip away from the leg-breaking gaps that plunged between them. On the best days, Mags and I would climb the trail until it emerged from the pine trees, and sit together on our rock at the side of the path, looking over the trees at the mountains and boulders I used to explore with Dad. On other days, like today, exhaustion and pain made a short stroll around the loch a battle of wills, or held me in bed, my mind screaming, and we didn't walk at all.

What had started as having to leave weddings a bit early had become having to call my understanding boss at the warehouse in York to apologise that I'd be late again, as I waited for the handful of painkillers I'd swallowed for breakfast to kick in enough that I could manoeuvre out of bed. Eating was an excruciating necessity, and frequent blockages contorted and shut down my intestines, leaving me writhing in agony, for hours, on the bathroom floor. Most days, when I got home from work, I only just managed to close the front door behind me before I collapsed on the hall floor and passed out with exhaustion, Maggie hungry and desperate for a wee, and staunchly by my side.

After years of being fobbed off, and months of leave-yer-dignity-at-the-door tests, the cause of all the pain had finally been diagnosed as widespread moderate-to-severe Crohn's disease, an autoimmune disorder of the intestinal tract. My body was attacking itself, causing inflammation, scarring and deep ulceration throughout my intestines. At the same time, I was diagnosed with another autoimmune disease, an inflammatory arthritis, which explained the merciless attacks on my muscles, joints, tendons, organs . . . Anything was fair game. Inflammation trapped the nerves in my back, sending bolts of pain down my legs when I stood, sat or moved, and the skin on the soles of my feet crawled with an unbearable itch which tested my patience beyond its limits. One winter, I stood barefoot in the snow for an hour, watching my feet turn blue, enjoying the relief of the numbness.

Despite our move to Aviemore, life and all its routines carried on as normal. In the evenings, Chris lay on his recliner watching box sets, while Maggie and I lay together under our blanket on the couch. Maggie kept my feet warm and I tucked her back in against the draught, and we'd both conk out.

'You said you'd watch this with me.' Chris was increasingly frustrated with my endless tiredness and lack of energy.

I stirred myself, and started the long, painful process of standing up. 'Sorry, I'll try to stay awake. Do you want anything from the kitchen?'

When we'd first moved from York to Aviemore, in December 2010, we'd landed in the off season, and although Chris had work lined up, finding a job proved impossible for me. At a loose end, and floundering, I was very happy when a well-timed email arrived from my good friend Pam, at Edgar's Mission, in Melbourne. Pam desperately needed a hand for a few months, and I really needed Edgar's Mission. So, in February, Maggie went to her gran and gramp's house for an extended holiday and I left the Scottish winter behind and spent three months in the Australian summer, doing all the things I remembered and loved from when I was there before, helping to take care of the rescued farm animals who called Edgar's Mission home. Through March and April, along with Pam, I was mum to four newborn orphaned goats – Magpie, Sooty, Richmond and Frankie – who were born into this world on the slaughterhouse floor, as their mums stood in the kill line. I tried not to think about that too much, as those thoughts tended to grip tight and hold on when I did. Instead, I focused on being a goat climbing-frame and an auto milk-dispenser, on call any time of day or night. The orphaned goats were delightful and full of the joys of being alive, and I adored them.

Although I always had to be near enough to a toilet, and some days needed strong painkillers to take the edge off, at

Edgar's, I found energy I didn't know I had. I got up at sunrise every morning, looking forward to what surprises the new day would bring. I barely noticed the time go by between stepping out of my old dilapidated caravan into the first sun of the day, and falling back into it, eighteen hours later, hardly able to keep my eyes open, a fulfilled exhaustion dropping me straight into a deep sleep.

I missed Maggie a lot, but once a week, I called Mum and Dad to get an update on her adventures, and I often got texts from her, telling me what she was up to on her walks. On Wednesday nights, Pam and I had a film night in the kitchen, a cat dozing on each chair, us on the floor. I'd usually only make it to the end of the opening credits before beginning to fall asleep. Pam would laugh, and put a blanket over me. It was hard, exhausting work, but it was bliss.

The end of May came round too quickly, and neither Chris nor the airline were willing to accept any more excuses for putting my departure date back again. As Pam dropped me off at the train station in Melbourne, the implications of my flight home went unsaid. Parked on double yellows, we kept our farewell pragmatically short. We hugged and I swung my rucksack on to my back. I didn't want to leave. I loved Pam and Edgar's and everyone who lived there.

'OK, so, Lex. Do you want a job at Edgar's? I'll help you get citizenship.'

Taken unawares, I stared at her.

'Think about it. You don't have to answer yet. I'm going to miss you big time, Lex. Right, gotta go. Love you. Take care.'

Pam was always busy, her life one never-ending to-do list, facing one difficult decision after another, one success after another, sleep often an optional extra, every day challenging and exhausting. She used all of herself – and more, if she needed to muster it. I had experienced that life and I wanted it. But although I loved Pam and Edgar's, did I want to follow someone else's path? What was I capable of? And though my heart and soul were at Edgar's, Maggie wasn't. Standing alone and bewildered outside Southern Cross Station, in front of me shimmering glass rose up from the pavement into the heat, dividing the paths that led towards two very different futures.

Arriving home in the early summer, I found it easy to get a couple of part-time seasonal jobs. In the evenings, I worked on the checkouts in the town's supermarket, and in the mornings and early afternoons, I worked as a receptionist in a Thai spa. The wee cabin in the woods that housed the spa was peaceful, and I enjoyed being there alone while the owners travelled or visited their family. It was an antidote to the exhausting cacophony of the supermarket, which was often a confusing and overwhelming challenge for my foggy brain. It was also small, so it was easy to find handholds, on my worse days, as I hauled myself from desk to treatment room and back again. A few hours in the afternoon, between the two jobs, was enough time to do housework and go for a walk with Mags, sometimes getting the chance to lie on the bed and stare at the ceiling, crying, for half an hour, before cycling down to the town for a shift at the till.

It was a mild late-summer evening, and I'd finished my shift at the supermarket and used the last of my energy to cycle home up the ski road. Exhausted and in pain, I parked my bike in the porch, closed the door and collapsed on the floor. The mat that declared 'Welcome' was ironically unwelcoming. The damp, muddy hessian scratched my cheek and the cold of the wooden floorboards seeped through my cheap nylon uniform. Maggie had heard me arrive home and took her spot, loyal and worried, by my side.

The season was drawing to a close, and I only had a few more shifts to go, but I had nothing left. Hope and joy were distant memories lying lifeless beneath the pain, exhaustion and frustration. Motionless, I stared at the wall. I was fed up of it all – the tiredness, the loneliness, the greyness, my failing marriage, the never-ending pain of my illness. I couldn't remember if there had ever been colour in the world, but even if there had been, it felt like there never would be again. The future was only ever going to be the same as today: a vast, bleak, futile, pointless nothingness.

I couldn't remember getting the knife, but I must have taken it from the kitchen drawer. My mind slipped in and out of functionality as it twisted and contorted, going one way then the other, sometimes moving too quickly to hold on to a thought, then grinding to a halt in an infinite, empty, heavy nothing. I needed out, and there was nowhere else left to go. I reached out and held Maggie's paw with one hand. The knife lay limp in the other.

You can't even do this right . . .

I looked into Maggie's eyes and my cheeks flushed with shame. I turned away.

Just a bit harder . . . just dig it in . . . three . . . two . . . one . . .

I'd lost my grasp on the slippery slope, and there was only one way to go now. There was only one way to end the pain. Lost in the darkness, Maggie's warm tongue on my face startled me. She was worried. I looked back at her, confused and anxious. I knew I loved her more than it felt possible to love someone, and I knew she loved me back, and I wished I could feel that love. She nudged my elbow with her nose. Tears stung my eyes as, ashamed, I slipped the knife into my pocket. 'You hungry, darling? Come on, let's get yer toast.'

A few days later, the rain finally relinquished its grip on the summer. Making the most of the fleeting sunshine and warmth, a group of us from the supermarket went to the local, the Old Bridge Inn, for a few drinks after work. Lost in the laughter and the booze and the summer evening, I ignored my phone ringing in my bag, knowing it would be Chris, and knowing the implications. After we got kicked out at closing time, we ended up across the road on the picnic benches, working our way through our accumulation of pints. It must have been gone two a.m. when I finally got on my bike and wobbled home along the cycle path. I crept into bed, trying not to wake Chris. It was a relief when he left for work early the next morning when I was pretending to be asleep.

Hearing the door of the spa open the following morning, I walked through from the back room. Chris stood in reception. My heart jumped.

'Where were you last night?'

'I was out with the folk from work. I texted you. They asked me if I wanted to go to the pub after work. I wasn't that late.'

I knew I'd been late, and I knew I hadn't gone home when I said I would. Adrenaline flowed, and my guts trembled. Years of miserable deterioration and dawning realisations had led to this moment.

'I was out looking for you! You didn't answer your phone. You didn't even come to bed when you got home.'

'I was checking Facebook . . .'

'Alexis, do you want to be in this marriage or not?'

I looked down at his feet and took a deep breath.

'No . . . I don't. I can't . . . Chris, you know this has been coming . . . Things have got really bad . . . I can't anymore. There's nothing left.'

Guilt, shame, relief.

Silently, Chris looked at me for a few moments. 'You're making a big mistake,' he told me, and turned and walked out the door.

I left the marriage, taking Maggie and a few odds and ends with me, and, because the house was tied to Chris's work, I was homeless. Mum and Dad offered to turn their conservatory and dining room into a living room and bedroom for me and Mags, so we could live with them and they could take care of me as my health deteriorated. I appreciated my folks' kindness and support a lot, but they understood why the thought of being so dependent made me want to flee the opposite way.

To make things easier all round, Maggie went to live with them for an extended holiday, and they gifted me my independence in the form of a bright green, three-door, eleven-year-old Rav 4. It was old and undesirable, as far as cars go, but I loved it. Along with a sleeping bag, a few changes of clothes, a book and a couple of carrier bags of things from the life I'd just left, I moved into the Rav.

Over the next few weeks, I lived in a travellers' hostel in Aviemore, sometimes slept in my car or on friends' couches, hooked up with a new set of acquaintances, and drank as much as I could, as often as I could. I gleefully lurched from a four-a.m. session outside the inn, to work, to horrible legal divorce stuff, to work, to another four-a.m. session. Me and my new friends from the hostel had parties in the Rav in the car park across from the hostel when it was booked up and I'd nowhere else to stay, and my best friend Karen came up for a few days to make sure I was keeping my shit together. We had a friendship that had aged and matured for fifteen years, and she knew what to do. She joined in with my nonsense, made me laugh like no one else could, and drank about as much as I did. It was all exactly what I needed emotionally, but it was a stupid way to treat a body already under attack and struggling.

I really missed Maggie, but I got regular hilarious texts from her, letting me know what she was up to on her walks.

Hi Lexis, I tooked Glan to the loch tooday, I was playin in the water wiv a big stick and I shook my head and Glan got all wet. Love Maggi xxx

*

33

Every couple of weeks, if I was up to it, I'd drive south and Mum, Dad and Maggie would drive north, and we'd meet in the middle, in Pitlochry. We'd have a car picnic and a stroll through the fallen leaves; I'd cram two weeks' worth of doggie cuddles into a couple of hours and make promises to Mags that we'd be together again soon.

It was getting darker and colder, and too much living on fumes was burning me out. Still, I slowly began to experience a return of the positivity, energy and enthusiasm I'd found in Australia, and I was ready to resettle and rebuild. Dad had just come into a fairly hefty inheritance from his uncle, William, whom we all called Wull. I'd spent a lot of my childhood on his sheep farm, sitting on his knee, thinking I was driving the tractor, and helping to bottle-feed the lambs. Ever supportive, my parents offered me some of the money to buy a flat in Aviemore. I gratefully accepted the chance of that independence, even if, financially, I was unrectifiably, and shamefully, dependent.

Maggie and I gathered up our few belongings and moved into our new home together on 11 November 2011. Maybe the colour was coming back, and maybe I could build a life for us. Maybe there was a future.

CHAPTER THREE

Twelve Days of George

The first snow of the winter arrived as December hit its stride. It was a bit later than usual, and determined to make up for it. The inefficient storage heaters in our flat had already been turned up full for a few weeks, and condensation pooled on the damp windowsills. High up, inland and far north, Aviemore had winters that were thuggish, relentless – and welcome, as the town's winter economic survival relied on snow hitting the mountains and skiers hitting the slopes. If ten degrees below freezing and thigh-deep snow was your thing, this winter was looking like a good one.

The last few winters had been especially bad; in 2010, the main arterial road up to the Highlands, the A9, had been blocked by snow that drifted well beyond the capacity of the snowploughs that were supposed to patrol and clear it. Snowed in and with temperatures hitting minus twenty, skiers had been forced to enjoy more holiday than they'd planned; as supplies started to run out, news of possible helicopter food-package drops spread round the town. I enjoyed the drama of Aviemore winters.

Where we lived – a low-rise block of flats at the south end of the main street – was quiet and far enough away from the shops and restaurants. The pine woods crept down the hill that loomed over and around the flats, blocking out a lot of the light and making the building a bit dark and damp, but Mags and I loved our wee home and we were nestling comfortably into the furrows of our new routine. My overall feeling in those first weeks of living there was gratitude; I'd only been homeless for a few months, but it had been long enough to miss time spent in my own company and to get a bit tired of using the wee green Rav as a wardrobe, kitchen, storage cabinet, bed and nightclub.

Free to find out my own taste in decor, I discovered that I really liked mismatched cushions, too many soft throws on the sofas, fairy lights on anything I could pin them to, and a windowsill overfilled with pot plants from the reduced-to-clear section of the supermarket. I didn't have the energy or money to put colour on the painted-to-sell magnolia walls, but I was filling the flat with pretty things in reds, blacks and bright greens, and the little dots of fairy light warmed and wrapped around us when we got back from our walks smelling of the cold and shaking off the wet snow from our coats.

When Chris and I had first arrived in Aviemore, I'd got in touch with Mandi, who ran the local dog rescue, to offer help. At the time, there wasn't much I could do practically – one dog was 'enough' – but we'd kept in touch and I followed the news about her dog rescue on Facebook. Idling away the hours one morning, a post caught my eye. I picked up the phone and called her immediately.

'Hi, Mandi. That old Lab you've just posted on Facebook . . . Bloody hell . . .'

From what the care worker who had found him had told Mandi, we knew that George was being kept in a shed and that his elderly owner had debilitating health issues, including dementia. As the man's health had deteriorated, so had his ability to look after the dog, who was now fourteen. He'd spent the last four years in a shed with no door, even in winter, ageing, aching and alone, with no bed and no company. Lying in the dirt, he'd watched life going on around him and without him. And, as he was often forgotten at mealtimes, he was usually hungry, too. Perhaps now there was something I could do.

'Could he come to live with us, Mandi? Do you think he'd get on OK with Mags?'

'Aye, I think he's used to other dogs. Are you sure, though? I don't think he's in a good way, Lexy. He might not have long, but I've nowhere else for him to go; all my foster homes are full.'

'Can we give it a go, see if he'll settle here? I cannae bear it, Mandi, the thought of what he's been through.'

'Right, let's get this old man a home.' And with that, Mandi started making arrangements to go and get George.

I sat on the arm of the sofa, panic rising, trying to make sense of what I'd just done. George was going to come to live with us, I was going to fall in love with him, and he might die. Pre-emptive grief pounded in my chest.

I lifted myself up. There wasn't time for this. Maggie was napping belly-up on the rug by my feet. 'Hey, Mags. Listen, sweetheart, someone's coming to stay.'

Later that afternoon, snow peaked high against the kerb as I pulled into the car park of the cul-de-sac where Mandi lived. Standing beside her, his head held low, was an old black dog. As I got out of the car, I watched as he started to lumber across the snow. His coat was thick and wavy, and the black had faded to greys and whites around his nose and cloudy old eyes. Slowly, he creaked across the car park, determination propelling his rigid, hunched body towards a small outcrop of grass, where he could lift his leg and maintain his dignity. He sniffed at a discarded wrapper lying in the snow, and started making his way back towards Mandi. When he reached her side, he wobbled to a stop.

'Bloody hell, Mandi.'

'It's bad, Lexy. Really bad.'

It was starting to snow again. 'Hi, darlin'. What's going on, eh?' I crouched down beside him. Swaying slightly on unsteady legs, he slowly examined my hand and turned his head towards me to put a face to the smell. I brushed the snow from his coat and felt shoulder blades that were far less padded than they should have been. His fur was thick with dust and grime, and calloused skin had taken its place where he had rested on the dirt floor. 'Oh, son . . .' I took his face in my hands and kissed the top of his head, blinking back tears. I stood up. 'Come on, handsome man, shall we get you home?' He looked up at me and wagged his tail.

Back at the flat, I sipped my tea and watched from the sofa as Maggie cheerfully welcomed George to her home. They sniffed their way around the living room, George following safely behind her, taking in this new world. When he was bathed and towel-dried, I could see he was delighted to be clean. It had taken four shampoos for the water to run clear in the shower. 'Look at you, mister!' I said, admiring him. 'You're so shiny, and you smell like coconuts.'

Hearing my voice, he walked over and rested his chin on my knee, looking up at me, wagging his tail. Surprised and delighted at how quickly he'd accepted me as his friend, I leaned forward and cradled his head in my hand, gently stroking my thumb across the top of it, sweeping the grey hair down around his eyes. I kissed his nose and massaged my fingers into the thick wavy hair around his neck, rubbing his tight muscles. He sighed and closed his eyes. I could feel tears start to well. He'd wanted for so much – food, a bed, a home – but what he really wanted, what he longed for more than anything else, was love. For someone to notice him, to care about him, to massage his aching body, to hold him and make it better. He'd waited so long for a friend, and despite the years of sadness and loneliness, he was desperate to love someone back. Wiping my face on my sleeve, I roused myself and stood up. He didn't need any more sadness. 'Did you enjoy that, hey? Come on, auld man, let's get some dinner in you.'

He followed me to the kitchen and watched as I prepared his food. Missed mealtimes flashed into my mind, the waiting and the gnawing hunger, the bowl that never came. I looked down at this wobbly, creaky old dog, waiting so patiently for the food that I could see he desperately hoped was for him. I wanted to fill him to the brim with food, warmth and love. 'Here you go, darlin' . . .' I put his dinner down in front of him. Slowly, he emptied the bowl and licked it clean.

'Was that good, aye?' Belly full, George stood in the kitchen doorway. I knelt down on the rug and he nudged his head against me. I folded my arms over and around him, and nestled my face into his warm, soft fur. I couldn't even imagine what his reality had been for the past four years. What had he thought about, as he looked out of his shed? What had he felt, as another day turned dark and he closed his eyes to sleep, his bed the same dirt he'd slept on the night before? How did he bear the bitter, bone-aching cold?

Four years alone in a shed. 'Oh, sweetheart . . . I cannae even imagine.' I massaged his neck a bit more. He moaned, and slowly melted on to my knee. I bent forward and kissed his fur, and he kissed me back, right on the nose. He'd lived for so long without any affection. How had his heart remembered how to love?

It was getting late, and it had been a big day. 'Come on, son, it's time for bed.'

I'd made a bed of thick fleece blankets for him, next to Mags' duvet, in front of the heater in the living room, and left a wee bone-shaped, dog-treat 'sweetie' on his pillow. I wanted him to be as comfortable as he could possibly be, now. 'Here, look! This is your bed, George, all cosy and warm. C'mere, I'll help you in.' He sniffed the blankets and paused, like he was trying to remember what he was supposed to do. He started pawing at the thick red fleece on top and nudging it with his nose. For a few minutes, he dug, spun and rearranged. Satisfied that his bed was nudged and dug to perfection, finally, he eased himself down. Mags had settled in her bed next to him and rested her chin on the side, watching us. As his broken old body nestled into the softness, his eyes closed. I kissed his head and tucked a blanket in around his back. 'Night night, darlin' man. Sleep tight.'

That night, for the first time in a very long time, George drifted to sleep in a warm bed, with a full belly and a friend by his side, in a home with a door.

The next morning, George woke early; from my bedroom, I could hear his long toenails tapping around on the laminate floor in the living room. Bleary eyed, I wandered through. A good sleep had worked its magic. He was standing waiting for me at the living-room door, tail wagging, eagerly looking up at me, trying to tell me something.

'D'ye need a wee, son?'

Coats on, we made our way outside. Stairs were a challenge his creaky bones could do without, so I scooped him up at the top and deposited him gently at the bottom. The grey clouds had dispersed, and under a clear sky, the three of us shuffled through the fresh snow. Wrapped up against the cold in Mags' spare winter coat, George wobbled his way along the grass verge that bordered the large field beside our flat, enthusiastically hoovering up the smells.

I watched him as he made his way from sniff to sniff. Life's natural decay, indifference and too many brutal winters had visibly taken their toll. His rickety legs swayed and trembled under him, and his back was hunched and stiff. He had an appetite, but not the appetite of a healthy, vibrant dog. His mind was willing, though, and his spirit flickered on, especially in his nostrils.

As he sniffed his way round his new stomping ground, I called Mags' vet, Gaby, and booked him an appointment for later that day. The coward in me knew there was a good chance I was going to find out something I didn't want to know.

At the vet clinic, George had some blood tests and X-rays, to see if we could get an idea of anything that was going on. While we waited on the results, we went to find out what sniffs Grantown-on-Spey had to offer, and slowly pottered our way round the block. When we got back, George wobbled in beside me, tail wagging, and Gaby gently delivered the news.

'It's not good, Lex. His liver is in a really bad way, and his kidneys aren't great.'

His X-rays showed that years of arthritis had fused his spine, his hips were disintegrating and his organs were starting to fail. He was already dying when we met, and the damage hadn't happened overnight. He'd been in a lot of pain for a long time.

'We need to control his pain,' Gaby said, 'but with the way his liver is, the medication is going to put him into liver failure.'

The words sank to the pit of my stomach. 'Is there nothing we can do, Gaby? There must be something we can do to help him. We have to . . . He needs to have more time.'

'I'm sorry. The damage is already done. The only thing we can do now is take away the pain and make him comfortable.'

Shock and anguish took my voice. This wasn't right, it couldn't be right; he'd waited so long, and now he was safe and warm, and he had a home and a family who loved him. I was desperate to make up for what he'd been through for all those years. Swallowing back tears, I braced myself to ask the question I didn't want answered.

'How long, Gaby? How long does he have?'

'He's in a bad way. Maybe a couple of weeks. Maybe less.'

Kneeling beside him, I massaged my fingers through the thick wave of black fur around his neck and touched my forehead to his. My heart ached.

'Are we talking days?' I asked.

'Probably. He's not got long. Take him home and make him happy. You'll know when it's time.'

I don't remember our journey home. The future I'd hoped George would have had evaporated in front of us. All those miserable years he'd waited for this – for love and friendship, for someone to notice him, for his own home. For four years he'd waited, and now he was only going to have days to know what it was like to be loved. It couldn't be this unfair, it just couldn't.

Over the next couple of days, Mags and her Lab-shaped shadow quickly settled into a comfortable ease, sharing sniffs and napping side by side in their beds, in front of the heater. George was basking in the relief provided by the hefty amount of pain medication.

While winter blew around us, in our cosy wee flat, the three of us huddled up together on the sofa. Mags was sprawled out on the rug, snoring and keeping my feet warm, and George had tucked himself into a ball beside me, his chin resting on my knee. I rearranged the blankets covering his back, and he edged himself closer to my leg, nuzzling in. I was trying hard to hold on to every happy moment, trying not to think of the darkness on the horizon ahead of us. Delighted by my friend's newfound joy, struggling to accept that he was going to die, and lost in the coming grief, I had no idea how I was supposed to feel.

By Christmas Eve, we had spent five lovely days together. Even in that short space of time, he was looking more padded and his eyes were brighter. Watching Mags and George together, they looked like they'd known each other for years. I'd already planned that Mags and I would go to Kilmarnock to spend Christmas with Mum and Dad, and they were glad to have another guest to share their table. It would be a long drive south, and it wasn't uncommon, at that time of year, for snow or an accident to close the road for a few hours. Sure enough, a snowdrift at the Drumochter Pass paused our journey. George and Maggie were sleeping on their duvet in the back, and every now and then, I'd see a sleepy head appear in my rear-view mirror, glance out the window to check our progress, and disappear back down, satisfied that there was still plenty of nap time left. 'Tough life, hey, you pair?!' I laughed, and turned back to my book as we waited for the snowploughs to do their thing.

We arrived late on Christmas Eve. Dad helped me unload the car, while Mum put the kettle on and Maggie excitedly showed George round her holiday home, helping him navigate the garden, kitchen and the cat-food stations, where there was a chance they might get lucky.

'You said he's not been used to being in a house? He doesnae seem bothered at all.' Dad and I watched as George explored the hallway, sniffing and shoving his nose into delicious nooks, cheerfully wagging his tail.

'He's amazing, Dad. I don't know how he is the way he is. He's a really happy guy.'

Once the tea had brewed, Mum and I sat down in the living room for a blether. We chatted about George, and I filled Mum in on his story. 'It's not fair – it's just not. He's such a nice guy. He loves his life so much. He's waited so long for this. I cannae bear it, Mum.' I was struggling to keep myself together.

Suddenly, the lights flickered and the whole house went dark.

'Oh, bloody hell!' Dad yelled from the kitchen. 'He's peed in the bloody plug socket!'

'Hey, George! It's Christmas! Come on, you've got presents to open.' Excitedly, but with no idea what he was excited about, George unfolded himself as fast as he could out of his bed by the radiator in the hallway. 'Come on, pal. It's yer first Christmas! Out for a wee, then it's present time!' Pushing away the sadness, I smiled down at him. *First. Not last.*

The five of us gathered round the tree in the conservatory. While we had our tea and toast, Maggie rooted through the piles of presents, looking for any that showed promise of being edible or squeakable. Stuffed full of bright, colourful parcels, hanging under the tree were two stockings, labelled *Maggie* and *George*.

'Awww, George, look! You've got yer own stocking!'

Cheerfully, he looked up at me, eyes full of wonder, panting with excitement. He had no idea what was happening, but whatever it was, it was good. It was the best.

Between Mum, Dad and me, we'd amassed quite the collection of presents for the auld man. Squeaky toys, chew bones, biscuits and a stylish new winter coat of his own. While Maggie ripped into her parcels, spitting out bits of soggy wrapping paper and excitedly investigating each new toy, George lay with his pile of parcels between his paws, looking from me, to Mum, to Dad, back to me.

I knelt down beside him and started to rip at the corners of the paper. 'Och, auld man, is it all a bit confusing? Here, look – like this.'

We laughed as he looked from his pile of presents, to us, to Maggie, back to his presents. He knew he was making us laugh, and he it was loving it. *My family.*

Parcels opened and excitement simmering down, Mum made them both a Christmas dinner, and they stood, side by side at their bowls in the kitchen, looking ridiculous wearing the paper hats we'd pulled down over their lugs. This was a meal that demanded total concentration to savour all the delicious new and surprising tastes. George licked his bowl clean, except for the lone Brussels sprout that sat dejected in the bottom. He gave it one last disgusted sniff and walked away.

'Do you not like those, auld yin? Me neither.' I followed behind him as he wobbled up the hall. 'Here, gimme that hat. Look at the state of you!'

After lunch had gone down, Dad, Maggie, George and I went for a potter around the golf course. When we got home, George found the best spot in the house, in front of the fire in the living room, and he dozed, occasionally opening one eye to watch his family spend the rest of the day as we'd spent every other Christmas: reading our new books, moaning about how much we'd eaten, and falling asleep in front of the telly.

'How was that, pal? How was your first Christmas? A bit confusing, eh? Yer face, with your presents ... Aw, you just loved it, didn't you?' I blethered to him as I tucked him into bed. He was tired out, ready for sleep. It had been such a good day and he'd loved every second. His first Christmas, with the best gift: spending it with his family. *His last Christmas*. A surge of grief washed over me. Sniffing, I whispered in his ear, 'I love you, auld man. I love you so, so much.' I kissed his nose, gave him one last sweetie and took myself to bed.

It was my first festive season since separating from Chris, and Dad was coming up to spend Hogmanay – New Year's Eve – with me, so I wouldn't have to be alone. On the drive home, we stopped off at some woods to stretch our legs. Looking dapper in his new coat, George explored yet another new place, filled with new smells.

It was bitterly cold and grey, a real depths-of-winter kind of day, and we shivered as we walked round the small loch, cracking the thin layers of ice as we traipsed through the muddy puddles.

Suddenly, I stopped in my tracks. 'Where's George?'

He'd been right behind us, padding along, following his nose, but now he was nowhere to be seen.

'Shit, Dad, where is he? I'll start walking back, you go down into the woods.'

Splash.

There he was, in the loch, doggy-paddling his way across it, looking absolutely delighted with himself.

'Oh, bloody hell, George! It's freezing! What the hell are you doin'?'

Cold be damned, this old dog was having the time of his life.

'Typical bloody Lab.' Dad laughed as George made it to the other bank and we fished him out. Adventure over, we bundled him into the car, dried him off, cranked the heaters up and tucked the duvet round his back. He looked very pleased with himself.

'Yer some man, George – yer some man.'

Almost as soon as we got home, I started to notice George slowing down. My heart ached as I saw his eyes grow more tired with each day that passed. He was still up for his walks and he didn't seem to be sore, but he was losing something. His spark was fading.

It was New Year's Eve and Dad had gone down to the shops to get some wine for later.

'Come on, son, lunch time,' I called through to George from the kitchen.

Nothing.

'George? You OK? Do you want your dinner?'

I walked through to the living room, where he was lying in his bed. Something was different.

'Hey, son, what's the matter?'

I knelt on the rug beside him and he looked up at me, weary.

'Let's see if we can find something you like, eh, darlin' man?'

I got his bowl and a spoon, and started trying to tempt him with his favourite food, but I could see even the thought of it was making him feel nauseous. Holding him, I could feel something starting to slip away.

'I love you, George. Please, not yet . . .'

Sick with worry and racked with doubt, I called Mandi.

'How will I know, Mandi? How will I know when it's time?'

'You just will. He'll tell you. And remember, it's better a week too early than an hour too late.'

Around four p.m. I'd gone to bed to have a lie down, as another wave of tiredness and pain took hold.

'Alexis . . .' Dad was calling me from the living room, and his tone sent a shudder of dread through me.

Shit, no.

George was standing by the door, his head hanging low, looking utterly miserable. He'd been sick, and a couple of pools of watery bile spotted the floor in front of him. Fear coursing through me, I lifted his lip. His gums were tinged yellow – jaundice: one of the signs that Gaby had warned me about that meant his liver was failing. It couldn't be. It was too soon.

You'll know when it's time.

I knelt down in front of him and lifted his head. His tired eyes met mine and I saw. His light had gone out.

Sobbing and distraught, I went into the hall and called Gaby.

'Oh, Lex,' she said. 'OK, bring him in.'

It was too soon. It was too cruel. I screamed, threw my phone at the wall and crumpled to the floor.

As Dad drove us to the vet clinic, I sat in the back seat with George, his head resting on my knee. He was fading fast. He'd been sick a couple more times and his legs were struggling to hold his weight, as his liver started to shut down and toxins flooded his body. I stroked his head and face, and whispered to him, comforting and reassuring him.

'I'm here, son, I'm here . . .' Every few minutes, he opened his eyes and looked around, confused and worried. 'It's OK, son, I'm here. Rest, darling. It's going to be OK, I promise.' I could hardly breathe.

He was too weak to walk, by the time we got there. The grey, washed-out light of the midwinter afternoon was fading as I gently lifted my pal from the back seat and carried him into the surgery. Every step was torment.

Gaby was waiting for us at the door. 'In here, Lex. Everything is ready. We'll make this quick and gentle for him, I promise.'

'Is there nothing we can do? Nothing at all? Medicines? Anything?' I pleaded, knowing it was futile.

My head dropped to my chest as grief grabbed my heart and suffocated it. The future George had waited so long for was over, and it had only just begun.

Kneeling on the floor of the consulting room, I laid George down and rested his head on my lap. He was barely awake, and he was fading quickly. Sobbing, snotty, gasping for breath, I wrapped my arms around him and burrowed my face into his fur. It was warm and soft, and it still smelled a wee bit of coconuts. I wanted to pause time.

'Just keep holding him and telling him you're there. Keep talking to him. I'll give him a sedative first. It's going to be just like going to sleep.'

'Twelve days, Gaby, he's only had twelve days.' I couldn't imagine anything could feel worse than this moment. 'I'm here, son, I'm here,' I said to George. 'I love you so much, darling man. I love you so, so much. I'm here . . .'

The needle emptied into his vein, and his breathing began to slow. A few seconds later, his heart stopped. He was gone.

Outside, families mingled in the town square, preparing for their New Year's celebrations. Empty, hollow, I walked slowly to the car and got into the passenger seat. As Dad drove us home, I turned and looked unseeing into the darkness.

When the bells finally rang to tell us a new year had come, I was lying in bed, Mags in her usual spot, keeping my feet warm. *Twelve days*. He'd waited so long for those twelve days. Had he been happy? Had I made his last few days good enough? I rubbed my eyes, replaying them in my mind. He *had* been happy. He'd been really happy. He'd had twelve days of pottering, sniffing and friendship. Twelve nights in a warm bed, in a home with a door. I couldn't change what he'd gone through before, but right at the end, he'd known twelve days of love.

I turned over and tucked the duvet round my back.

'Goodnight, auld man. I love you.'

CHAPTER FOUR

Somewhere Nice to Die

'Is that good, Mags? You enjoying yer paddle?'

She was pottering around, entertaining herself in the shallows of the Green Loch, investigating floating sticks and pausing every so often to catch the sniffs on the breeze. I watched her from my perch on the smoothed, weathered remains of a long-dead tree on the sandy shore, and I was smiling at this happy moment when, catching me unawares, a fresh vein of grief lurched up from my gut. Watching Maggie enjoying herself in the water reminded me of George's impromptu swim on our walk at Christmas, and how pleased with himself he'd been. The pangs of grief still took me by surprise. I'd be out walking with Mags or folding a blanket that I'd once tucked round George's shoulders, and they'd erupt without warning, just as raw and overwhelming as they had been that first time, kneeling on the floor of the vet's surgery, holding his body.

Sometimes I managed to nudge my mind in a different direction and focus on how happy George had been in his last few days. It rounded the edges of the pain a bit, but three months on, the grief and injustice of his life and death still hurt like hell. Maggie had loved having a pal, and she missed having him around as well. The auld man who couldn't stay for long had left a big space in both our lives.

At the same time, the Crohn's was still draining me. The simplest task took everything I had, and I was becoming less and less inclined to find the will to do even basic household chores. Too often I'd find myself creasing my face in disgust as I dropped yet another tub of half-eaten mouldy hummus into a bin that could've done with being emptied a week ago. Too many days I'd scuttle down the stairwell embarrassingly late in the morning, Maggie desperate for a wee, wearing the jammies that I'd probably still be wearing when it was time to go back to bed again.

Both of the jobs I'd had the year before had finished, and the progress of both the Crohn's disease and the inflammatory arthritis made getting another job really difficult, though I did have a short-lived stint as a cleaner at the hostel where I'd lived for a few months the year before. I was in a lot of pain, and I was lethargic, ashamed and frustrated, mainly with myself. For the most part, Mags and I were each other's only company, and it was Mags that kept me from sinking into my bed and probably never getting out of it again. Aye, I was often a bit late dragging myself down the stairs for morning wees, but every day, no matter the pain or the tiredness or the what's-the-point-ness, I *did* manage to drag myself out of bed, down the stairs and on through the rest of the day.

Bored and restless, but too weak to live a normal life, I spent a lot of time online. Early in the year, I started getting involved in helping to save stray dogs from the pound, sharing their posts and donating to help them, when I could. I'd had no idea that stray dogs were still killed in dog pounds, and I was horrified when I realised that it was happening all over the UK, to hundreds of dogs every week. One day, I found myself on a Facebook page of a 'pound puller' group that helped to save as many dogs as they could from being killed. This small group of dedicated folk networked for rescue spaces and foster homes, organised transport for the dogs they saved and tried to raise the money needed to pay for it all. From the photograph, the bewildered eyes of a Staffie stared back at me.

This lovely lady is Roxy. She's a friendly girl who likes a fuss. Roxy was left in a lay-by, and she isn't chipped and has no ID tag.

Roxy, like any other stray dog, only had seven days to be claimed or found a rescue space before she was killed. She had one day left. There were pages of photographs of other strays in exactly the same situation. Chihuahua, Staffie, lurcher or springer spaniel, every one of them was confused and terrified, wondering what the hell was going on after being dumped on the street or left tied to a lamp post. Their pitiful pound-issue mugshots captured a pleading sadness as they looked out, bewildered, from behind the bars of death row.

I couldn't bear it. I felt totally helpless, and what they were going through started to really get into my mind and haunt me. That night, I lay awake for hours thinking about Roxy, alone and afraid in her kennel, her time almost up, booked to be killed the next day. I woke up in a panic, too frantic even to put my glasses on before pressing the phone to my nose to check notifications and see if a miracle had arrived in time. Thankfully, for Roxy, it had, and I sank back into the pillow in relief. But I knew that, for many others, miracles didn't happen, and whenever I thought about this, I'd lie and stare at the ceiling and cry, unable to understand why we had to live in such a hellish world.

In March 2012, I saw two photographs on the Facebook page of a group I'd been helping. Several miles apart, but with similar sorry tales to tell, Ri and Annie had each been abandoned and taken to their local dog pound, another two unwanted dogs among thousands. As usual, there wasn't much information, but in her write-up, Ri was described as a timid, red and white Staffordshire bull terrier, who was nearly three years old and had two days left before she would be killed. She was microchipped, so the pound had called her owners to let them know she was there and that she was going to be killed if they didn't go to collect her. 'Yeah, that's fine,' they'd said. 'We don't want her back – just kill her.' I couldn't comprehend it. If Maggie had been missing, I'd have taken the world apart trying to find her.

Annie was a middle-aged tan cross-breed, probably a bit collie and a bit Staffie. Her teats sagged, a reminder of her life as a puppy factory, and she was very underweight. The information about her said she was very fearful and in pain, and there were signs that she might be aggressive towards other dogs.

I knew that, with pound kennels and rescues around the country full to bursting, there weren't many options for Ri and Annie. It was hard enough to find rescue spaces and homes for healthy, young, well-balanced dogs; for two older, traumatised, possibly aggressive dogs, it was almost an impossibility. But it was rescue space or death for them, and time was running out.

George had left a light on. Aye, there were shards of grief wedged in my heart which felt like they wanted to split it right open sometimes, but if that was the price for his twelve days of family and love, so be it. The pain wasn't just worth it, I was actually glad I was feeling it. It was really hard to miss someone so much, but I'd still rather have known him than not. I knew that having another two dogs in the flat would be a huge challenge, but I wanted Ri and Annie to have a chance at life, like George. Anxious, and a wee bit exhilarated, I messaged their pound puller, Shelle, to offer them a foster home.

On a Sunday morning in late March, with just hours to spare, Ri and Annie left the kennels in Essex where they'd both been brought to start their long journey north. Dogs often have to travel a fair distance to get to their rescue spaces, and the transportation is usually done in a relay system, with a few drivers working in a tag team to split longer runs, meeting for handovers at prearranged locations, usually service stations. It's a delicate process and there is a lot of room for things to go wrong. Which is exactly what happened this time.

It had been a horrendously worrying day, and at about midnight, it became clear that things had gone so badly wrong that I'd have to go and collect the dogs myself from the vet clinic in the middle of England where they were being held overnight. At two a.m. I set off on the nine-hour drive from Aviemore, knowing it would be a slog. I left Maggie at home and had arranged for a neighbour to pop in and feed her in the morning. It was a stressful and tiring journey anyway, but another flare-up was rapidly draining my batteries. During a stop, I was standing in the queue of drivers waiting on their caffeine high when reality dawned. I was on my way to pick up two dogs, one or both of them might be dangerously aggressive, I already had a dog to care for, and some days I could hardly get out of bed. Somehow, I was going to have to find a way to make this pantomime work in a first-floor, two-bedroom flat.

Almost twenty-four hours after I'd left, I pulled into the car park outside my flat. Ri and Annie were as confused and shocked as me, and they weren't the only ones wondering what the hell was going on and what was coming next.

'You've bitten off more than you can chew,' my neighbour told me gleefully, as she saw me coaxing two anxious, worried dogs, one by one, up the stairs.

Aye, you might be right.

In the first few traumatic and very stressful days, Ri chewed, peed on or clawed every single item of furniture in the spare bedroom. One afternoon, as we came in from our walk, a bad memory must have stirred in her as I bent to pick up the free local newspaper from the mat, and her belly hit the floor in fright.

After a few walks, it became clear that I would have to be very careful with Annie around other dogs. Because of her issues, the only safe space I could find for her was in a large crate in the small kitchen. Most of the time, she'd shrink to the back of her crate as I squeezed past to get to the cupboard behind it, but sometimes she'd launch herself forward, growling and smashing her bared teeth against the metal. As I got to know her, I realised that it was all coming from the years of neglect, abuse and living in fear that she had suffered, and although I was wary, I knew she didn't want to hurt me. She just didn't know what else to do. Life had made these defences necessary and she wasn't going to forget them quickly. The insides of her ears and the pads of her paws were a raw, itchy, infected, scarred mess. She had a few scars that looked a lot like cigarette burns, and there was a small diamond-shaped scar carved into her side. Left untreated for so long, these chronic ear and skin infections were driving her half-mad, and I was trying, but struggling to get on top of them. I got the feeling that Annie hadn't known peace for a long, long time. Both Ri and Annie were highly traumatised, destructive and unpredictable. It was understandable, but it was very stressful – for them, for me and for Maggie.

Perseverance, patience and stubbornness kept us going, and, as the months slipped by, thankfully the dust started to settle.

Overnight, my once-idle days had become full; I had to walk everyone separately, and, after finishing one round of down-the-stairs, through-the-woods, back-up-the-stairs for each of them, I had just enough time to get a cup of tea before starting back at the beginning again. It was exhausting, and trying to put one foot in front of the other while the Crohn's depleted every bit of my energy was almost impossible some days. But, like Maggie, they needed me, and hard as it usually was, I knew that dragging myself out of bed was the best thing for me, too.

When I wasn't out walking, I tried to split my time between them as best I could, to make sure they were all getting enough company and affection. It had turned into a lovely summer, and we filled the warm, pleasant days pottering around the field or the woods at the back of the flat, and going on jaunts further afield, into the wilds, in the wee green Rav. It took some doing, but with a bit of consistency and a lot of willpower from us all, Ri, Annie, Maggie and I started to settle into something resembling a contented routine.

On midsummer evenings, I'd sometimes take the twenty-minute drive along the winding, single-lane road to Loch an Eilein. Standing on the banks of the loch, I watched Maggie and Ri paddle in the still shallows, making ripples that spanned out across the water. I enjoyed the long summer days of the far north, the days that weren't clear about where they ended or began. Looking across to the ancient ruined castle on the island in the middle of the water, still visible in the suspended dusk against the steep and thickly wooded far bank of the loch, it felt like we had stepped into a different world. I loved it.

Over the summer, Maggie and Ri had become good pals. Though she was a lot more relaxed and content, Ri was still anxious and had the occasional wobble when she misread Maggie's intentions and assumed she had to get her defence in first, but it was never serious. Her huge Staffie smile and heart full of love were a tonic, and she had a delightful bounce to her step and shine to her coat. In typical Staffie fashion, she had to be as close to me as she could possibly be, give me as many kisses as she could possibly fit into a day, and, in bed, her wee bald Staffie belly was my toasty, comforting foot and ankle warmer. We were in love.

Annie and I had also come to adore each other, but we tested each other's patience to the limit. Years of neglect had taken their toll, but underneath it all, Annie was full of love – and, like George, despite everything, she hadn't forgotten what to do with it. She had big brown eyes and black eyebrows that she used to good effect for her varied repertoire of facial expressions. She still had her issues, and I still had to live like I had a pet velociraptor, but together we were finding the things that helped her forget what had gone before, and looking for the things that made her come alive.

One afternoon, on our walk, Annie and I had discovered one of those things. I tried to find places that were remote and away from other walkers – and, specifically, other dogs – and we'd found a beautiful spot by a river that we both loved, hidden down a wee track through the pine trees, away from the hordes in the park. It had become a regular spot for us to enjoy, and while I sat on the bank, leaning against an old pine, reading my book, Annie paddled and sniffed around, enjoying her freedom. I had just opened my book and got settled in when I heard a commotion coming from the river. Alarmed, I jumped to my feet. Annie was in the middle of the river, head down, back legs sticking straight up in the air. Panicking, I ran to the edge of the water, but as I watched her, I could see she was snuffling around and digging in the stones on the bottom, back legs flailing, the black tip of her tail wagging arcs of water as she scrambled around. She wasn't in distress at all, I realised; she was stone fishing, and she was loving it.

Seconds later, she came splashing back to the surface in a snotty, breathless, joyful mess, with a huge stone in her mouth. Grinning, she hauled herself up out of the water and deposited her treasure on the bank. I'd never seen anything like it. She was clearly delighted with herself.

'Go on, Annie, do it again!' It was a joy to see, but she didn't need any encouragement.

Annie spent the summer refining her technique. Her dives became ever more ambitious, getting longer and deeper, and she was rewarded with bigger and better treasures. She developed a categorisation system, too. Each fishing trip, she'd have three piles, and every stone had to be allocated to one of them: the closest pile was for your run-of-the-mill, average-Joe stones; the next one, a bit further from the water, for your slightly more prized good-but-no-cigar stones; and, furthest away, a pile for the Kings of Stones, the Boulders among Stones. She carefully deposited each one in its proper place, and gave me a quick, thrilled side glance as she ran as fast as she could back to the water to do the whole thing all over again. Even as we got towards the end of the stone-fishing season, and the cold water started to turn her pink after a few minutes, she'd go for as long as I'd let her and I'd often have to drag her away shivering. Every time, the biggest stone – the Stone of the Day – came home with us.

My plan had always been to try to find new homes for Ri and Annie, but near the end of the year, I decided that we were going to stay together. Ri was a great lassie, full to the brim of Staffie goodness. I had fallen in love, and so had Maggie, and I couldn't bear the thought of life without her. It had taken Annie and me a long time to trust each other, but we'd got there, and we'd become really good pals. She was starting to find peace, but she was still a bloody liability around other dogs, and I wasn't going to uproot her, or pass her and her issues on to someone else. So, difficult as the balancing act was, I decided that she was staying put, too. It had been a difficult and challenging few months for all of us, and there were tears of frustration in the harder times and tears of joy when the breakthroughs came, but we'd muddled through and we were going to keep muddling through.

With a job still out of the question due to my ridiculous body, I was doing whatever I could to help the pound dogs, and getting to know the people who worked hard to save as many as they could. They were always struggling to raise the money to pay for the dogs' transport and vet treatment, and I wished I could do more to help them, but I barely had enough money to meet our own basic needs. I started thinking. Was there a way that I could raise some money to help the dogs? Sometimes they were dying because there was nowhere for them to go, but sometimes it was because there was no money to pay for them to get to a safe place, which seemed like even more of a betrayal. I didn't have much money, but I did have plenty of time, so I put out the feelers to the folk who were helping them and asked if a reliable source of donations would help to save more dogs. 'Yes,' was the unequivocal answer. Before I had time to stop myself, I had a plan.

I had no experience of fundraising, no idea what I was doing and no confidence, but a stubborn streak runs through the women in my family and the fledgling idea wasn't going to be satisfied until it had a chance to take off and see what happened. I used the couple of hundred quid I'd saved up to buy a web domain and hosting package, and got to work. I didn't know where to start with building a website, I didn't know how professional fundraising worked, and my body was a disintegrating wreck. Yet somehow, between me and my battered old laptop, by February 2013, I was ready to launch Pounds for Poundies. The plan was that each dog would have their own page, with a photo, a brief description and the date they were due to be killed. I'd log their donations on their individual pages and I'd use that money to pay for their transport, emergency kennelling and vet treatment. I hoped it would make it easier for rescues to offer them spaces, knowing that at least some of their costs would be covered. I had no idea if it was going to work, but if it could raise even a couple of hundred quid a month, it would help a few dogs on their way to a safe future.

A few days after I'd made the leap and pressed *publish*, I watched in astonishment and bewilderment as my phone pinged with donation after donation. In the first week, Pounds for Poundies raised more than £10,000, and, within a few weeks of launching, I applied for official charity status. I was confused, delighted and terrified. Very quickly, it took over my life, and I worked on it all day, every day. As it grew, more pounds became involved, and within a few months I was adding dozens of dogs a day to the website and raising and distributing thousands of pounds every week to help save them. Even with my good friend Iona's dedicated help, it took at least twelve hours a day to keep it all running, and a good few nights a week, there were frantic one-a.m. transport payments, as we rushed to get someone off death row. I was stressed and overwhelmed, but I felt useful again and I was overjoyed that my plan was working. I'd forgotten what boredom was and life felt a lot more colourful – maybe there was some point to it, after all.

Mags, Ri and I wandered through the woods, shafts of light cutting through the treetops. The air had changed in the last few days. The autumn chill had arrived on the breeze and the world was responding: leaves were losing their grip on branches and the red squirrels were starting to hunt for hidden spots to keep their winter treasure-troves safe. I kicked at the leaves as I chatted to Dad on the phone, glancing over at Maggie and Ri to check what they were up to.

'I got the blood results back, Dad. It's what we thought. It's starting to go for my liver.' The chemotherapy drug I'd been given to try to batter my immune system into submission was starting to have serious side effects, and my latest fortnightly blood-test results showed that my liver was starting to fail.

'What happens now? Is there something else they can give you?'

I could hear the concern in his voice. I hated the worry my disease gave him and Mum.

'I don't know, Dad. I'll ask the nurse at my review, next week. But I cannae keep taking this stuff.' I was often stuck between a rock and a hard place; the medication to try to stop my body attacking itself was causing devastating, life-threatening side effects. I was hanging on by a thread and I was running out of options, time and will.

By the end of 2013, the Crohn's was constant and gnawing, doubling me over in ceaseless spasms, and eating was torture. Anything solid felt like crushed glass, cutting and grinding its way over the raw, inflamed tissue, and even water hitting the ulcers and abscesses in my stomach caused stabs of pain that made me want to scream. When it became too painful to eat, three gruesome apple-flavoured nutritional drinks a day kept me alive, sometimes for months at a time.

The inflammatory arthritis had also had a very productive year, every flare-up finding yet another target for its rage. My muscles, joints and tendons would swell and ache, and sharp, hollow pains shot up the inside of my bones. At one point, I was taken to the local A & E with a suspected broken foot, but it turned out that my body was attacking my toe joints with such ferocity that it just *felt* broken.

*

'Come on, Mags, darling. You can do it.' I was struggling with the stairs up to the flat, and they were starting to be a bit of trouble for Maggie, too. She was about seven, now, and it was undeniable that her joints were feeling the strain. Since George died, I'd started to dwell on thoughts of Mags' death. I'd watch her sniffing, exploring or lying asleep on the rug, and think about what it would be like when she wasn't there anymore. I'd swirl the thoughts round and round until grief overtook me, and I'd spend the next hour sobbing and miserable over something that hadn't even happened. I tried to shake away the thoughts and just enjoy our moments together, but they never fluttered far off their perch before coming back down to land.

By November, I could barely get out of bed. Every morning felt like I was stepping onto an exhausting, uphill treadmill that was never going to end. Only the flat was keeping me in Aviemore, and even that was starting to become difficult for Maggie and me.

'A garden would be handy,' remarked Dad, as he helped me and Mags down the stairs during one of his visits to see us.

'Aye, it sure would,' I agreed. The thought of having our own secure space, where we could be free and not worry about meeting other dogs, was a sweet, tantalising dream.

'Why don't we have a look?' he suggested. 'See if there's somewhere out there?'

Being winter, the housing market was slow, but within a few weeks, I'd been to view a little wooden-shingled cottage, set in half an acre of woodland in Ballindalloch, near the Spey Valley, a bit further north from Aviemore, right in the heart of Scotch whisky country. It was in the middle of nowhere and the garden was more than big enough to keep Maggie, Ri and Annie entertained on my worst days. It was perfect, and with Dad's help, I put in an offer. It was accepted, and in January 2014, Mags, Ri, Annie and I packed our bags and moved to our wee cottage in the woods.

The cottage had two bedrooms and a bright living room with a small wood-burning stove. The kitchen was dated and the wallpaper was peeling off in places, but the living room and the sunroom looked out over the garden and down to the woods, with the River A'an sparkling between the trees below. Pheasants, woodpeckers, owls, red squirrels and deer also called this bit of the world home, and at the most, we saw maybe a couple of dozen cars pass us in a day. It gave us some much-needed peace in our lives, and from the second we walked in, it felt like home. On our first morning there, I opened the door to let Annie out by herself – no harness, no lead – and she looked up at me in disbelief.

The breeze was carrying the promise of warmer times to come as I stood on the porch, sipping my tea. I watched Mags sniff her way around the garden, tail bouncing, nose twitching and lugs flopping, taking her time on what had become her daily morning perimeter sweep. When she'd finished, she plonked herself down on a mound of grass in the middle of the garden, surveying her new territory, nose to the wind. I was so grateful for this new, peaceful way of life and the freedom it had given us. We'd been through a lot, the four of us, and now here we were, hidden away from the world in our wee cottage in the woods. I winced as the tea hit my stomach, the first spasm of the day. The four of us had finally found our peaceful place, and – although it went unsaid – it was a lovely place to fade away, and die.

CHAPTER FIVE

Six Weeks

I stepped back, out the way of the grey snow slushing up on to the pavement, as the coach pulled into the stop. Mags and I were bundled up against January's cold, but there was a chill in my bones. The door slid open and the folk arriving from Glasgow started to make their way down the stairs, bracing themselves as they stepped into the snow. Mum was somewhere in the queue. She was coming up for a few days to visit for my birthday, and to help me drive to the hospital to get the results of some recent tests.

I shook my head and rubbed my eyes, trying to break through the foggy tiredness that always hung around. Mum and I hadn't seen each other for a few months, and I wanted to be cheerful for our hug and catch-up on the drive home. The lead wrapped round my wrist tugged me forward. Delighted, Mags had spotted her gran at the top of the stairs; forgetting all her manners, she rushed forward to greet her, past the legs of the people waiting to get on the coach. Smiling, I watched the two of them, so excited to see each other – Maggie wrapping herself round Mum and almost knocking her over, Mum bent forward, trying to grab Mags for a kiss. They adored each other.

'How was the journey? Did you get yer cup of tea?' I asked, as we hugged. We always joked about Mum getting to ride for free, courtesy of her old fogey's bus pass, on the posh Gold Bus, the first-class coach service from Glasgow to Aviemore, with its complimentary Irn-Bru and cups of tea. As we pulled away from our hug, I was surprised to see that she was crying.

'Mum, what's wrong? You OK?'

'You . . . you don't look well.'

Seeing me in the flesh had taken her by surprise. I was used to myself, and hardly noticed the hollow greyness of my face and the scrawny body that looked about fifty years older than it was.

'I'm OK, Mum. I'm just tired,' I reassured her, obviously lying. 'Let's get to the car; it's freezing.'

It was nice to have company, and Mum was determined that she was going to look after me. Life had become really difficult, and I was grateful to her for taking care of things for a few days while I worked away at Poundies, slept and indulged in some distracting box sets. I had an appointment at the hospital the next day to see the inflammatory bowel disease nurse for tests, and to get the results of a recent MRI, and Mum wanted to come with me. We knew it wasn't going to be good news, but I'd heard it all before. The disease was progressing, the medication wasn't working, I was more ill than I had been at the last visit . . . The usual. I had long since accepted life trapped in a malfunctioning body that was irretrievably wired up wrong.

'Alexis? Hi, nice to see you.' The nurse was standing in the doorway of his consulting room, smiling at me like an old friend. I shuffled up the corridor, hunched over and dragging my feet, Mum walking beside me, carrying my coat and bag. The nurse was a kind and understanding man, and he made me feel comfortable and reassured about the ins and outs of life with Crohn's. I eased myself into the chair by his desk.

'Right, Alexis, we've got the results of your last MRI.'

Mum, sitting next to me, gripped my hand.

'It's not good,' the nurse said. 'The pain you've been feeling in your right-hand side is because the disease has got worse. It's become stage three; it's started to fistulate.'

Over the last ten years, I'd learned a lot about Crohn's, and I'd suspected this was coming. Relentless inflammatory attacks on my intestines had finally managed to eat through the intestinal wall and out the other side, into my abdomen. A large part of my intestine was an inflamed, diseased, squishy mess that was full of holes, barely held together by scar tissue.

'The only way we can fix this is to operate and cut it out, but your blood results aren't great. You're too weak for surgery and it would be too risky. I'm sorry.'

Mum choked on a sob and squeezed my hand, but I wasn't remotely surprised that my body had been condemned like a defunct old boiler. I'd already guessed that I was dying.

For a few reasons, I had decided that I didn't want to take the big-gun drugs I'd been offered as the next and ultimate stage of treatment. But interestingly, a few months before, I'd met someone who also had severe Crohn's, who had been successfully using plant medicine to treat it for a few years. She had put herself into remission and she was healing her own once-condemned body. I'd been thinking about it since we met. Was there another way I could try to treat and heal my diseased, depleted body?

'I've been doing a lot of research into cannabis oil,' I said to the nurse, 'and I want to give it a try to see if it might help.' I knew he couldn't advise me, but I had to be up front with him about what I was intending to do.

'Right, aye . . . Well, whatever you're going to do, do it quickly. You've got about six weeks.'

It was the day before my thirty-fourth birthday.

'I'm OK, Dad. But, aye, it's still sore.'

Dad called every evening to make sure I was still standing. It had been twelve weeks since Mum and I had been to the hospital, and, though I was beating the odds and hadn't keeled over yet, I was really struggling. In the months since, I had used all the energy I had to research and find things that might support my body and help it start to heal. Years of not being able to eat or digest food properly had left me dangerously malnourished, and I was trying to find ways to start building myself back up again. I'd visited a herbal doctor, who prescribed me some remedies to help soothe the inflamed tissue and take the heat out of my overkeen immune system, and Mum and Dad had filled the cottage with supplements, juices and nourishing food. I was trying, but I wasn't feeling much – if any – improvement. It felt like I was standing on the edge of a volcano, taunting its rage with an ice cube. It was a daily battle to hold on and keep going.

'What about the oil?' Dad asked. 'Is that doing anything yet?'

I'd started taking the cannabis oil on my birthday. I was scared and apprehensive, and still taking tiny amounts that were far less than the medicinal dose.

'I've been taking it, Dad, but it's not doing anything.' My disease didn't usually scare me, but I was losing the will to fight it and I was already living on borrowed time. 'What if it doesnae work?'

I could see the car parked in the lay-by at the end of the dirt track that ran up the side of the golf course, following the river down the valley. Enjoying her walk, Annie was investigating some dried leaves, happy and relaxed and taking her time on the bright, hopeful April day. Another wave of nausea lurched up from my guts and I doubled over, retching. I stumbled to the side of the path to throw up, but nothing came; it had been days since I'd been able to eat anything. I tried to stand up. Dizziness whited out my vision for a few seconds, and my legs and bowels gave way. I crumpled in a humiliated heap, sagging on to the dry, withered undergrowth at the side of the path. Annie looked at me, worried. Bracing myself, I tried to stand up, but my legs were having none of it. I looked along the track: we were still a couple of hundred metres away from the car. I closed my eyes and took a deep breath. My body, mind and spirit were crushed. I sat on the verge, with Annie beside me, self-pity, fear and humiliation washing down my face in hot, frustrated tears. If this was life, I didn't want it. I was fucking done with it. I took another deep breath, turned myself around and started to crawl on my hands and knees towards the car.

Back at the cottage, I staggered through the front door, into the hallway and through to the kitchen. Leaning on the worktop, I opened the cupboard and grabbed the small bottle of oil, still almost full. I unscrewed the cap and took a big swig. I cleaned myself up, limped through to the bedroom, collapsed on to the bed and let the exhaustion drag me into sleep.

Promising spring sunshine flowed into the bedroom as I opened the heavy velvet curtains. Maggie and Ri were still in bed, blinking awake. I wandered through to the kitchen to put the kettle on while they did their morning stretches.

'Come on, you pair, out for yer wees.'

Yawning, they meandered through from the bedroom towards the front door, stopping on their way down the steps to get a sniff of what the day had on offer. Sipping tea at my usual spot on the porch, my eyes followed Mags as she diligently performed her daily perimeter sweep. She stopped to sniff at some pioneering daffodils who had stuck their heads up to see if the time had come for them to sound the spring alarm. The sun was tempting me to stay out a bit longer, so I sat down on the step of the porch, gazing up along the garden to where Ri lay flat out, sunning herself in a warm spot. I paused. *Hang on a minute.* I had almost finished my tea, and I didn't feel anything. Nothing. Not a twinge, not a spasm. Why didn't I feel like I'd just swallowed a mug of crushed glass? Where was the pain?

The days went by. Although I often still ached, twinged and spasmed, the oil seemed to be giving me more and more moments of relief. Before, the pain had become so constant that it was like background noise, and I had got used to tuning all but the worst of it out. But now I was feeling what it was really like not to be in pain, even if only for snatched, blissful moments. I was sleeping much better, too, and though I still had some darker times, in general I felt much less like some dreadful unknown thing was about to happen at any moment.

Amazingly, not only was I eating, but, for the first time in almost a decade, I actually had an appetite. It came and went, but I was starting to enjoy some of the things I'd used to love to eat. Every day, I shoved vitamins, supplements, potions and beetroot juice into me, and although I sometimes had to strictly parent myself away from tea and toast towards something more nutritious, I was eating small, healthy meals almost every day. It was a revelation. After so long of understanding that eating equalled pain, I'd forgotten what it felt like to enjoy food or to feel better after a meal rather than worse.

'Alexis, hi, nice to see you! How are you feeling?'

Back at the hospital in May, I was seeing the nurse for a

check-up. It was my first visit since he'd gently told me I might not see spring. I strode into the consulting room, bursting to tell him how well I felt. Anxious, nervous and a bit excited, I hoisted myself up on to the examination bed.

'I'm just going to have a quick feel of your tummy, see what's going on,' he reassured me. 'I'll try not to hurt you.'

'On you go. It's fine. Prod away.' I smiled, relaxing on to the bed as he tapped and prodded his way round my guts.

'Does that hurt?'

I shook my head.

'What about here?'

It didn't hurt, not even a bit.

'I don't know what to say,' he stuttered. 'The inflammation is gone.'

'Yer looking not bad,' I told the mirror as I brushed my teeth. My cheeks were pinker and slightly rounder, and though I was still scrawny, I was starting to lose my freshly-dug-up look.

As spring unfurled, I was surprising myself by how far I could walk, and the dogs and I were discovering new and interesting routes that took us further up and down the valley. The grass was starting to reach skyward, and not only could I start the lawn-mower – an insurmountable challenge that had left me shouting and sobbing in frustration, the summer before – but I could mow the entire lawn in one go. I was delighted with myself. My batteries still discharged pretty quickly and needed a lot of time to recharge, but I was doing things that, just a few months before,

I never would have imagined I'd ever be able to do again. I ate lunch on the grass on nice days, read more and baked. I'd even adopted two turkeys, William and James, and my dream of offering a home to some rescued laying hens had come true. I'd been very careful to keep the dogs away from them at first, especially Annie, but our new feathered friends didn't seem to bother any of them. Miraculously, my spark was coming back, the bit of me that fired up all the other bits, and I felt light and free. I wasn't trapped on the inside, looking out, anymore.

I turned off the tap, dried my mouth and walked through to the living room to turn on the stereo. I was in the mood for a bit of a dance.

I stepped back, out the way of the puddle washing up on to the pavement, as the coach pulled into the stop. Mum was grinning down at Maggie from the top of the stairs, jacket over her arm, holding her book.

'So, did you get yer tea?' I teased as we hugged, almost tripping over Maggie as she wriggled around us and wrapped her lead round our legs. 'Aw, for goodness' sake! What are you crying for, now?'

'It's *you*! You look so well!' She smiled.

'Fancy lunch at the Mountain Cafe, Mum? My treat?'

CHAPTER SIX

Three Dogs, a Chicken and
a Sheep Walk into a Bar . . .

As the life force started to flow through my veins again, I finally had the energy to do something about the discontentment and loneliness that had been quietly gnawing away at me. I loved my new life in the cottage, being with the dogs, chickens and the turkey lads, and I was basking in the relief of not being exhausted and in pain anymore. But I was longing for someone to share it with, and I was a bit worried that I couldn't quite be trusted to hold life together competently enough by myself.

Given that I rarely left the house except for our walks or to go to get chicken food in Elgin, my chances of meeting someone in real life were slim to none. I couldn't think of another way of doing it, so – what the hell? – I might as well try to meet someone online. My profile – *I love dogs, chickens and going to watch Tornadoes take off at Lossiemouth* – hadn't had much success in the few weeks I'd been despondently, but addictedly, logging on to check for matches. I'd broken the dating ice a couple of weeks before, when I met someone for a few drinks in Glasgow, but the initial excitement had long since worn off, and the whole thing felt more like trawling estate-agent websites with £500,000 worth of criteria and a £100,000 budget than it felt like looking for love.

I'd been staying in Kilmarnock for a few days to celebrate my pal Karen's birthday. I'd brought Annie, Mags and Ri with me, as usual, as well as a chicken called Mary, because she hadn't quite been herself recently and I wanted to keep an eye on her. I wasn't ready to give up on the torture of dating just yet, and tonight I'd arranged to meet a guy for a drink in Ballater, a couple of hours south from the cottage, in the heart of the Cairngorms National Park. My original plan was that I'd leave Kilmarnock in plenty of time to drive home, drop off my entourage, make myself look presentable and head south again to meet him.

I was getting ready to leave when Clare, my friend from university, with whom I'd shared almost twenty years of life's laughter, frustration, joy and despair, texted to tell me that she'd just received some devastating news. Quickly, I changed plans. I would go and be with Clare for a couple of hours, get changed at her place, then leave in time to go directly to Ballater. I wouldn't be able to go home and drop the dogs and Mary off, but if I kept it to one drink and made my excuses, they'd be OK in the car for an hour or so. It wasn't ideal, but needs must. I got our things together, hugged

Mum and Dad goodbye, detoured to the supermarket to get cake and Kettle Chips, and set off to see Clare at her flat in Glasgow.

While Clare and I drank tea, ate crisps and cried, the dogs took it in turns to potter around in the back garden, while Mary clucked about helping Clare's toddling boys with their mud pies and gardening.

'Aw, shit, is that the time?' I said. 'I better go, I'm gaunnie be late for this bloody date . . .'

Of course, we'd lost track of time. I bundled my charges into the car, while Clare bundled hers into the flat. Standing outside her front door in the old, draughty, traditional Glasgow tenement, we held each other in a long goodbye-I-love-you-and-take-care hug.

'Right, I better go. Call me if you need anything, OK? See you soon.'

'See you soon. And drive safely – don't rush!'

Clare waved as, wearing the same clothes I'd had on yesterday, three hours away and already running late – and with three dogs and a chicken in tow – I set off for my date.

We were almost an hour north of Perth and making fairly good time. At Perth, I'd taken a different road from the one I usually took home, driving straight through the middle of some of the highest and most remote parts of the Cairngorms National Park. The route up through the mountains was narrow and dotted with passing places, and there wasn't much to distinguish between what was road, what was mountain and what was a sheer drop. Misty autumn rain swept in curtains over the scree slopes, washing grey across life's colour, and high on the slopes the sheep who roamed the hills were white blurs against their grey world. Mags, Ri, Annie and Mary were hunkered down in the car, bracing themselves against the twists and sharp corners, as the windscreen wipers slopped back and forth.

'You lot OK, back there?' A shiver ran through me, and I reached across to turn the heating up a few degrees. The bleak, cold, desolate landscape made me want to wrap someone I loved in a blanket. Rain splashed up over the windscreen from the puddles pooling on the road as we rounded a sharp bend and bounced over an old humpback bridge. As we pulled away from the bridge, I put my foot on the brake, frowning. Something had caught my eye. *Was that a lamb?* My sheep senses were tingling; something wasn't right.

I slowed to a stop and reversed into a lay-by. I checked the clock: it was just before six thirty. I had an hour until I was due to meet my date, and we were just under an hour away. Doable, just, if I was quick.

Opening the door, I braced myself for the cold blast and glanced both ways. Head down against the driving rain, I ran back along the road towards the bridge. A few sheep who were grazing nearby startled, paused for a second, and scattered up the hill into the mist. Through the rain, I could see a shape slumped against the old stones: a lamb, hunched over, soaked and shivering. *Shit.*

Trying not to startle him, I slowly walked closer and crouched down beside him. He looked around six months old. His head was hanging forward and his long black ears drooped over his closed eyes. He could barely hold up his head, and his nose was almost touching the wet tarmac. Gently, I put my hand on his back. He flinched, and turned his head away from me, towards the wall.

'Oh, sweetie.'

Even through his thick fleece, I could feel the bones of his spine, and he was swaying slightly on legs that were struggling to support his weight. He was soaked through, trembling with cold, and small whorls of sodden wool clung to his cold, pink skin. As I wrapped my arms around him, I felt the water from his fleece seeping through my shirt. A healthy lamb his age who'd never been near a human would have been halfway up the mountain by now. There was clearly something very wrong.

Gently, I lifted his head so that I could check his gums: they were sticky, cold and pale, which I knew were signs of hypothermia and dehydration, or potentially something worse. I had no idea how long he'd been there on the bridge, but he was in dire straits and I knew, if I left him there, he wasn't going to survive the night. In northern Scotland, where hill farms often cover thousands of acres, there was no hope of finding the farmer. I had two choices: leave him there to die, or take him home.

I stood up, wiping the dripping strands of hair back from my face and blowing drops of water off my nose as the rain hit my skin like needles. It wasn't that long ago that I had been the one collapsed at the side of a road, feeling rotten, helpless and hopeless. This little lamb needed warmth, a full belly and someone to carry the load for a while. He needed a friend. There was only one option.

'I know, son, I know . . . Wait here. I'll be right back.'

I jogged to the car and grabbed the dogs' towel and a blanket from the boot, moved Mary's crate over a bit on the back seat, and made sure Annie was securely seat-belted in the front.

'Bloody hell, lassies. Here we go again.'

Jogging back to the bridge, I was relieved to see him still barely standing in the spot I'd left him a few moments before.

'It's all right, son, I'm not gaunnie hurt you.'

He had no reason to believe me. I wrapped the towel around him and, frightened, he tried to wriggle free.

'Oh, darlin', I know. Try not to worry. I'm sorry.'

Holding him tightly, I quickly lifted him off the ground and cradled his body into mine. Helpless and dejected, he sank into my arms and his head fell against my chest. I kissed the soaking wool on the top of his head and nuzzled my nose into his fleece as the tears welled.

'It's OK, sweetie, it's gaunnie be OK.'

The water from his fleece was seeping through my jeans as I half-jogged, half-stumbled back to the car. Manoeuvring the door open, I heaved him up and across the back seats. He was under-weight, but in better days, I could tell he'd been a big, robust lad, and he was still a match for my upper-body strength. Blinking, eyes wide, he watched me as I climbed in beside him.

'I know, son, it's scary, isn't it? Try not to worry. Right, we need to get you dry.'

Mags and Ri were watching from the back, and, in the front seat, all Annie was missing was a box of popcorn. Mary, deciding that whatever was happening was not important and/or interesting, was head-under-wing asleep, or at least pretending to be. On the back seat, the lamb lay quiet and still. He was life-threateningly cold, and he desperately needed to start getting some warmth into his bones if he had any chance of surviving. Leaning over the gearstick, I turned the temperature controls and air up to full. As the warm air started to fill the car, I rubbed the towel over him, and little fibres of damp wool clung to my fingers. From experience – including the time when I almost lost my fingers to frostbite climbing the Cobbler, a spectacular peak in the Southern Highlands, having them saved by sticking them in Dad's armpits and screaming in agony for an hour – I knew I had to be really careful to raise his body temperature slowly and steadily, or risk causing more damage. Ideally, he needed direct heat, like a heat lamp, a hot-water bottle or body heat. Out here, in the bleak, desolate Cairngorm mountains, the only source of direct heat I had was myself.

In the back seat, wedged between a chicken and a sheep, I squirmed and wriggled out of my soaking jeans and shirt. My skin was cold and clammy, and rain and damp sheep had turned my shirt into a straitjacket. Trying not to upset him, I squeezed myself in between his woolly body and the seat. He barely flinched as I pulled him close and tucked Maggie and Ri's fleece blanket tightly round us. As I wrapped my arms around his freezing, shivering body, I could feel the cold start to seep into me, and he trembled and spasmed as his body threw everything it had at staying alive.

'Come on, darling, come on. Keep fighting . . .'

As we lay there, wrapped up together in the back seat, I imagined how scared, confused and worried he must be. In his six or so months of life, he'd probably only ever seen humans as they sped past in cars, and now he was inside a car, vulnerable, weak, not able to get away, trapped with a human who could have any intention towards him. Had I done the right thing?

For about forty-five minutes, we lay there together on the back seat. I whispered gently to him, trying to reassure him, my face burrowed into his damp wool. Aware of the time ticking by, I lifted my head to get a look at the clock on the dashboard: it was just before seven thirty, five minutes before I was due in Ballatar. *Shit.* I squeezed my hand under his armpit to check his temperature, and with great relief, I could feel a little bit of heat starting to build up. I checked his gums, and the faintest hint of life was starting to come back to them, too. I closed my eyes. *Thank you.*

'Right, darling, we better get moving.'

I shuffled myself out from behind him and wrapped the blanket tightly around his body. Stirring, startled, he tried to lift his head to see what was happening. He had a long way to go, and I needed to get him home and get some nourishment into him. I was pretty sure I still had some lamb milk formula in the house that I'd bought in spring, just in case of any newborn-lamb emergencies. But first, I had to go on this bloody date. Given that the poor guy had already driven two hours to meet me, I felt I had to at least show my face for half an hour, even though it was the last thing I wanted to do. I wriggled and grimaced my way back into my soaking, clingy, wet-sheep shirt and jeans as elegantly as

I'd wriggled out of them. Maggie, Ri and Annie – who had lost interest in this movie when it got to the boring, quiet bit – had settled down, and I let them out for a quick wee as I buttoned my shirt and squelched back into my boots.

We were still an hour from Ballater, and I had about thirty seconds to get there. Although I was notoriously and shamefully late for everything, on this occasion – at least to me – it felt justified. I just had to hope that my date felt the same way.

Back in the driver's seat, I leaned over to briefly check my reflection in the rear-view mirror. The light was dim, but I could see that specks of mud and blood – *blood?* – dotted my face, and my soaking, frizzy hair was scraped back against my head. What was left of my token application of make-up – a wee dash of eyeliner – was smudged and streaked. This, coupled with years of anxiety-induced obsessive eyelash pulling, gave my naked eyes the look of a mole who'd just woken up with a killer hangover. Starting to panic, I reached for my handbag to get my eyeliner. A wet strand of hair was pestering my eye, and, getting more wound up by the second, I lifted my hand to brush it away, bear-pawing myself square in the face and taking out a contact lens. *Awfurfuckssake.* Now I was a half-blind hungover mole who smelled like wet sheep and looked like I'd been living in the mountains for a year, rather than driving through them for an hour.

Fuck it.

I started the engine and – now with three dogs, a chicken and a sheep in tow – third time lucky, I set off for my date.

*

An hour and fifteen minutes late, and a fretful, wound-up mess, I pulled into the dark, deserted car park in a town that, on such a depressingly miserable night, felt almost as bleak and inhospitable as the mountains surrounding it. Cheeks flushing, I steadied myself and got out of the car, zipping up my ski jacket over my damp shirt, and walked to where my date was waiting.

'Hi. Sorry I smell like wet sheep,' I blurted. As opening lines go, it was a belter.

Self-consciously, we introduced ourselves and I started to explain what had happened.

'You should have just left it to die,' he interrupted. 'That's nature.'

'Are you fucking serious?!'

What the hell are you doing.

'Sorry,' I said. 'It's been a really long day . . .' Frantically back-pedalling, I smiled hopefully. 'Shall we find somewhere for a drink?'

Instinct was telling me to get myself and my ever-increasing entourage home, but I couldn't just bolt from the situation I'd created. My date had been patient, and I at least owed him a drink. The lamb was getting warmer and, feeling guilty, I figured half an hour wouldn't make a huge amount of difference.

'Sorry, but we'll need to find somewhere that allows dogs . . .' I was under no illusions about the limit of Annie's self-control, and it did not extend to being left unsupervised in a car with a vulnerable prey animal.

Thankfully, on a dismally dreich Wednesday night in September, there weren't many folk around, and within a few minutes, we found a hotel with a welcoming owner who was happy for us to sit in the foyer with Annie. Coming out of the drizzly rain, frozen to the core and in dire need of some warmth, I was grateful to see a fire burning in the hearth and an empty sofa in front of it. We got in a couple of drinks and a bowl of chips, while Annie sat people-watching on my jacket on the floor beside me, her leash tightly wrapped round my wrist. Whatever the poor guy was saying, I wasn't listening. I just wanted to get back to the car, check the lamb was OK and get him home.

He needs a name . . . Angus . . . Aye, that's nice. Angus.

As we fidgeted, sipped our drinks and made agonising small talk in between the long staring-at-the-floor silences and the using-Annie-as-a-conversation-filler moments, I noticed that the guy was slowly slithering down the sofa. While we scraped together things to talk about, he inched further and further towards the floor, until only his neck and head were propped up against the sofa cushion, while the rest of his body sprawled out across the tartan carpet and into the foyer. *What the hell was he doing?* He wasn't drunk; we were both drinking orange and lemonade. I glanced down at Annie, who looked up at me, eyebrow raised. I sipped my drink faster, feeling self-conscious, thinking of Angus, confused as hell. I wanted to teleport home, but I stuck it out as we finished our drinks, while he talked to his own nipples and I got well acquainted with the top of his head.

Finally, back at the car park, we said our goodbyes, each of us hoping that the other wouldn't be polite enough to feign an interest in arranging another go at that cringeworthy disaster. As he drove off, I checked on Angus and let the dogs out for their wees. Thankfully, the lamb was keeping his body heat and he seemed stable. I climbed in and closed the car door, sighing with utter relief that my date was over. Somehow, I'd turned up looking and smelling like I'd been living in a cave with three dogs, a chicken and a sheep, and he had *still* managed to out-weird me. There was hope for me yet.

Blinking awake, I started groggily trying to work out where I was and why I could hear hooves clunking around on the carpet. I turned over and reached for my glasses. Beside me, two big black ears framed the curious woolly face looking into mine.

'Oh, hey, Angus . . . Wow, look at you!'

When we finally got home last night, I carried him in from the car and the warmth had started to spread through his chilled body, bringing him back to life. I found the milk and a feeding bottle, and with the little bit of energy the heat had given him, he managed some dinner. I'd decided that the spare bedroom was the best place for us to get some rest. It was warm and I could sleep in the bed and keep a close eye on him through the night. The nourishment and the long sleep in a safe, warm place had worked their magic. From his bed in front of the radiator, he'd managed to stand up by himself, and the few black nuggets trampled under-hoof into the carpet showed that he'd been busy while he waited for me to wake up. He was clearly feeling much brighter, and by the look of it, he was wondering where breakfast was.

I swivelled out of bed and knelt down beside him on the floor.

'Feeling better, hey?' I wrapped my arms around him and nuzzled my face into his warm, dry wool, smiling with relief. 'You hungry, son?'

He blinked up at me, tilting his head. Surely, he should be scared of me – this frightening human thing, who had, to all intents and purposes, abducted him a few hours before?

'Right – breakfast time. You coming?'

I quickly got dressed and fed Maggie, Ri and Annie, and the bird folk outside. While I prepared his bottle, Angus wobbled his way around the kitchen with Maggie and Ri, who were just as accepting of our guest as they'd been the night before. Seeing how much he'd perked up overnight, I was feeling a lot more hopeful. But I knew there must have been a reason he'd ended up on the bridge like that, even if it had just been plain bad luck. I called the vet in Elgin to make an appointment for him to get checked over later that day.

'Right, son, let's get this into you . . .'

Smelling the milk, twitching his ears and licking his lips, Angus trotted behind me, back into his bedroom. At six months, he was too old for a bottle, but the milk would give him everything he needed, and it was easy for his body to digest. It was a relief to see him tuck into it so enthusiastically.

'Bloody hell, you made short work of that, pal!' I put the empty bottle on the bedside table and slid down off the bed and on to the floor. 'C'mere, you – gimme a cuddle . . .' I leaned against the bed and pulled him closer to me.

The warm milk was making him sleepy. It wasn't just his body that had taken a battering, alone on that bridge; just finding it in himself to survive out there must have taken all his will and spirit. He had a lot of healing to do, and another good sleep, on a full belly, and a rest from his worries, was the best place to start.

'Look at the state of you!'

Frothy white bubbles foamed in the dark wool around his mouth, in a little milky beard. Unable to resist the pull any longer, sleepy and content, he sank into my arms. I bent down and kissed the black curls on his head and pulled my fleecy shirt around us. The events of the day before had tired me out, too, and I was finding it as hard as Angus to resist a snooze. We had a couple of hours before we had to leave for his vet appointment. I leaned back against the bed and closed my eyes, smiling: what a difference twelve hours had made.

For a Thursday afternoon, the place was heaving, and the only parking space anywhere near the vet clinic was in a supermarket car park across the road. Until the day before, Angus's reality had been mountains, scree slopes and sheep. I found towns overwhelming enough, so I could only imagine how he'd feel about them. Cautiously, I opened the boot of the car.

'OK, son, let me get a hold of you . . .'

He was alert, but lying down, thankfully not looking like he planned on doing a runner. Carefully, I bundled him up and wrapped my arms securely around him, propping him up with my leg as I manoeuvred the boot closed.

'Right, let's go!' Rushing as quickly as I could while carrying thirty-five kilograms of sheep, I made my way across the car park, trying to avoid eye contact with shoppers pushing laden trolleys back to their cars. Angus was the most surprising lad; even among the traffic and noise and smells, which must have made him feel like he'd landed in another dimension, he didn't bat an eyelid. Balancing him on my knee, I opened the door to the vet clinic and we tumbled into the waiting area, only a couple of minutes late.

'It's OK, son.'

The vet had lifted Angus on to the table to examine him, and I stroked his head as she listened to his heart and his chest, and checked his gums. I wasn't sure, but he seemed more tired than he had this morning. Maybe it was the stress? Anxiously, I whispered to him and kissed his head as the vet tried and failed to find a vein so she could get a blood sample and run some tests. Angus was getting more upset, his eyes frantically darting to me, to the vet, to the walls.

'Oh, darling, I know, I know . . .' In the pit of my stomach, I knew something wasn't right.

'OK, I'm in,' said the vet, drawing a slow trickle of blood into a syringe. 'I'm going to give him some fluids, too; he's very dehydrated.'

Steadying myself, I wrapped my arm around his shoulders. He was trying to stand up, but he could barely lift his head before it was too much and he collapsed back on to the table.

'Try not to worry, darling. It's OK. We'll be home soon.' My stomach was turning. He'd been so bright this morning, guzzling his bottle and jigging about the bedroom, but my instincts were telling me something was seriously wrong. While the vet ran the tests, I knelt down next to Angus and tried to reassure him. He was breathing quickly, and his eyes were wide with worry. I kissed his wet nose and touched my forehead to his. 'It's OK, son. It's OK . . .'

Gradually, his breathing started to slow down. I was just easing myself to my feet as the vet opened the door, looking at a printout. I knew before she said the words.

'It's not good news, I'm afraid. His liver and kidneys are already failing, and his heart's not good. He's very malnourished. He's low on almost everything: potassium, calcium, magnesium.'

I wrapped my arms around him. 'Is he going to make it? Will he get better?'

'He's in a bad way. Whatever's wrong has been wrong for a long time. I'll give him some fluids and antibiotics to make him feel better, and some pain relief, too, just in case. I don't know what caused it, but I think the damage is already done.'

That morning, I'd started to hope that all that time he'd fought to stay alive, all the courage it had taken for him to keep going through the cold and the rain, the pain and the loneliness and the despair, that it had been worth it, and that he was going to get to live the life he'd hung on to despite everything. We'd known each other less than twenty-four hours, but I knew Angus wanted to live, and I'd hoped that I'd be able to help him do it. I stared down at the floor, as the life raft of hope drifted away.

'Hey, Angus. How you feeling, son? It's dinner time . . .'

Hearing me opening the door, he turned to watch me. His too-big-for-his-head browny-black lugs stood straight out from his warm, sleepy face. He made me smile. When we'd got home from the vet, the evening before, I'd made a bed for us in front of the wood burner in the living room, and we'd spent the night there, tucked up cosy on the duvet, drifting in and out of sleep. He'd been eating, not quite as enthusiastically as he had that first day, but enough to keep him going and to keep my hopes up a bit. With sleepy eyes, he watched me as I pottered around the living room, tidying up while his milk cooled. Outside, William and James, the turkeys, were threatening a lorry on its way to or from the distillery.

'D'ye hear that racket, Angus? That's gaunnie be you, one day, out there on that grass!'

I checked his milk on the back of my hand, took off my slippers and squeezed myself under the duvet beside him.

'Right, you, c'mere . . .'

I rearranged and straightened our bed a bit, and got him into position beside me, holding the bottle up to his nose, ready for him to start drinking. He sniffed at it for a few seconds and turned his head away.

'Come on, son, you need to eat. You need to keep yer strength up.'

I tried again, squeezing a little bit of milk on to his lips. He turned away: *Nope.*

I closed my eyes. *Please, no.*

It was starting to get dark. I turned on the lamp and the pretty lights around the bookshelf that cast dragonflies across the walls, and, manoeuvring around Angus, I stoked the fire and added another log. Maggie, Annie and Ri had had their dinner, and although they'd had to forgo their walks for a couple of days, as Angus's needs took over, they were content with a potter in their garden by day and a snooze on their sofa in front of the fire by night. I'd made some fresh milk for Angus, and while it cooled, I went outside to put the bird folk to bed.

Returning to the living room, I offered the bottle to Angus. 'Come on, son, just a wee bit? Please?'

He turned his head away. I put the bottle down and wriggled my way under the blankets. We were facing each other on the pillow. I gave him a few kisses on the fuzzy wool above his nose and he nuzzled into my neck.

'I love you, son . . .'

His eyes fluttered. He could hear me, but he was being pulled deeper and further away into a sleep he could barely fight.

'Are you sure you don't want any more?'

Mustering his strength, he opened his eyes, and as we lay together, looking into each other's faces in our wee cosy nest in front of the fire, he told me what I didn't want to hear. His spirit had tried, but it couldn't fix his broken, depleted body. His light had gone out. He was done.

I knew what it was like to be stuck inside a broken body, and I wouldn't wish it on anyone. I could be his cheerleader, and I could buoy him up and give him food and warmth and love and a warm bed, and make sure he wasn't sore, but the fight . . . that was his. If he didn't want to – or couldn't – fight anymore, all I could do was understand and accept, no matter how much I'd hoped. I put the bottle, still full, on the hearth and tucked the blankets around us.

Together in our warm bed in front of the fire, in the quiet of the night, we drifted in and out of sleep. Every so often, we'd stir, stretch and rearrange ourselves, and I'd stoke the fire and tuck the blankets round us. Angus was nuzzled into my neck, his warm, sweet breaths tickling my ear, and my nose was pressed into his warm wool, comfortingly soft and sheepy.

I think I always knew that our time together was going to be short. Whatever was wrong with Angus had been wrong for a long time, starting long before we met. But our paths had crossed – somehow – on that bleak, cold road. I couldn't change what had gone before, and I couldn't release death's grip on my new friend. I didn't have much power to change things in this world, but I could take cold, hunger and loneliness and replace them with warmth, a full belly and love.

As dawn broke, I stirred from my sleep. Angus was still cuddled contentedly in my arms, but his breaths had slowed down and I could feel that he'd drifted further away. He was getting ready to leave.

'It's time, eh, son?'

Ever so slightly, he stirred, and relaxed back into my arms. I kissed the thick black fuzzy wool on his head and stroked the soft bit on his ear, and together we lay in silence as the world woke up around us, and we waited for what was to come.

CHAPTER SEVEN

Ebb

'Wait, Mags, let me help you.'

Half-on, half-off the bed, Maggie looked at me. As unwilling as I was to accept that doing it by herself was a challenge too far, these days, I could see she was struggling. I scooped her into my arms and hoisted her up.

'Don't worry, petal, it comes to us all,' I reassured her. 'There we go. C'mere and I'll tuck you in.'

I wanted to ignore it and pretend it wasn't happening, but for the last few months, Maggie had been getting creakier as arthritis prowled into her bones. Her hips and knees were getting stiff and sore, and my heart hurt seeing her struggle to get up on to the couch and into the car. Not so long ago, she could propel herself on to the bed without thinking about it, but now, every night, I had to hoist her up and watch her ease herself slowly into her sleeping position, comfort not coming quite as easily as it used to. Even getting up from lying down was becoming an effort for her, and I winced as she heaved her protesting hips into action after a snooze in front of the fire.

She'd been seeing her vet, Ailidh, for acupuncture every couple of weeks, and I'd been giving her massages, which were easing her pain and keeping her mobile and comfortable. Though she was slowing down, she was bright and happy, she still loved her days in the garden and she was as enthusiastic as ever for her grub and night-night toast. I was adding supplements to her food to keep her joints oiled and I gave her medication every day to control the pain, but although her mind was still raring to go, it was clear that Mags' body was finding everything a bit of a strain, these days. Although there was no hiding from life's decay, I was hopeful that, with careful management and maybe a ramp for the car and a few other things to help her, she still had a lot to look forward to.

A few weeks later, I was doing some cleaning and watching her sniffing her way round the garden, when I noticed that she looked a bit swollen around her waist. A bolt of worry shot through me.

'Mags, c'mere and let me get a look at you.' Wrapping my arms around her, I felt her belly. 'Oi, sit still, you!' *Was that fluid?* Her abdomen felt like a water balloon. Why would there be fluid there?

As far as I could tell, everything else was normal. She was happily pottering about the garden, sniffing, exploring and sun-bathing – all the things she loved. She was eating with as much enthusiasm as normal, and she'd not shown any sign of being unwell. But something clearly wasn't right. I wanted to pretend I'd not seen anything and carry on with life as it had been a few minutes ago, but much as my cowardice and fear put up a good fight, I knew I had no choice but to find my courage.

'Love you, Mags.' I gave her a squeeze and left her entertaining herself in the garden, while I went to call Ailidh.

After a good check over, Ailidh couldn't find anything obvious, but it was a pretty bad case of ascites – accumulating fluid – and there were a few things that could be causing it. I didn't want it to be any of them. At a loss, Ailidh referred Mags for an appointment at Broadleys, a specialist animal hospital in Stirling, where they had the equipment to do more thorough diagnostic tests. If we had any hope of fixing it, we had to find out what was causing it.

A few days later, in the predawn darkness, I bundled a half-asleep Maggie on to her duvet in the boot of the car, ready for our trip to Stirling. I didn't want any of this to be happening, and I was absolutely dreading what they might find.

The day dawned into a bright, chilly morning, and, shivering, I zipped up my coat and helped Mags out of the car for a much-needed wee. Mum was driving up to meet us, to share the waiting and worrying, and we waved her into the car park as we wandered around, exploring the shrubs.

'Hi, darling girl! Come here and give Gran a kiss.' Mum was trying to be cheerful, but I could feel that she was as worried as me. While Mags did her wees and sniffed around at the smorgasbord of smells, Mum and I hugged and blethered about our journeys.

'C'mon, we better get in.' Mum nudged me. 'It's almost nine o'clock.'

Anxiously, I opened the door of the clinic and Maggie swaggered into the waiting room, tongue lolling, smiling at the receptionist, her proud, worried gran and mum following behind. Mags worked her charm as we chatted with the consultant who was going to do the tests, and by the time we kissed her big brown head goodbye and promised her we'd see her soon, she had already wormed her way into the hearts of the folk who worked there.

Mum and I spent the day in the Waitrose cafe near the animal hospital, drinking pots of tea and trying to laugh ourselves through the worry. But it was an agonisingly long day of waiting. Just after four o'clock, my phone rang: Maggie was coming round from the anaesthetic and doing well, and the consultant wanted to talk to us. Nervously, we drove back round to the hospital and took a seat in the large, busy reception. I closed my eyes, tired from the drive and the worry, and sort of hoped that I'd be in a different reality when I opened them again.

'Ms Fleming?' The nurse's voice startled me from my dwam. 'Maggie's ready to see you. Just through here . . .'

Mum and I jumped from our seats and quickly made our way across to the open door of the consulting room.

'Maggie! Oh, petal, it's so good to see you.' She was still a wee bit drunk from the anaesthetic, but she was delighted to see us. We wrapped our arms around her, kisses flying in all directions.

The consultant, a kind and considerate man, dimmed the lights to show us the images from some of the scans they'd taken. He told us that there wasn't anything significant in her abdomen, but something suspicious had shown up on the scan of her chest.

'I'm sorry,' he said, clearly understanding how hard it was to hear what he was telling us. 'She's going to have to go to the vet hospital in Edinburgh for more tests. Try not to worry too much. We don't know anything for sure yet . . .'

I looked at him, silent, blinking, as reality shifted around me. I looked down at Maggie, sitting beside me, sleepy and cheerfully looking into space.

'I'll make the arrangements, and we'll be in touch.'

I nodded. I was grateful for his kindness, but I didn't have any words. I knew, whatever the tests found, it wasn't going to be good news.

Back at the car, I helped Maggie into the boot. Neither Mum nor I knew what to say, so we hugged and set off on our long journeys home.

I stood and smiled as I took in the view at one of my favourite places – Findlater Castle. The dilapidated, once-magnificent castle sat high on a cliff overlooking the North Sea, and its treacherous nooks and crannies had enthralled me since I was a toddler.

I'd been coming here with Dad since I was wee, on the promise that I never told Mum about all the dangerous things I got up to there. Today, Maggie, Ri and I had come for a special day trip.

A few days ago, my worst fears had come true. Tests at the vet hospital had confirmed that the suspicious mass that had showed up on the scans was a tumour on Maggie's lung. The only option was long and dangerous surgery, and tomorrow morning, I had to take her to the hospital for her pre-op check, to prepare her for the operation the day after.

The castle was a special place for me that I wanted to share with Maggie . . . from a safe distance. Mounds of wet, muddy earth slid down towards what used to be doorways and windows. For years, Dad and I had hidden the photos of me standing, arms outstretched, in an ancient doorway, nothing but a good pair of soles and a good bit of luck between me and the edge, the sharp rocks lying waiting in the surf, a hundred feet below. I had much more appreciation for Mammy's worry, these days.

Back at the car, I arranged a duvet on the grass and laid out our picnic. The clouds had cleared, and we'd found ourselves a sunny spot that was heating us up nicely. Mags was nose to the sky, catching the scents on the breeze, while Ri sat on the duvet and vibrated, trying her hardest to keep the fountain of Staffie excitement from overflowing.

'You having fun, lassies?' I smiled down at them, tickling the glossy fur on top of Mags' head and running her soft, velvety ear through my hand.

Thud thud.

The timing of her operation was so unfair. Almost miraculously, over the last few days, the fluid had cleared by itself, and Mags was feeling pretty chipper. Her latest session of acupuncture had given her some welcome relief from the stiffness that plagued her hips, and she'd enjoyed our walk along the cliffs. She loved going to new places, and for as long as we'd known each other, Maggie and I had enjoyed finding interesting walks and exploring them together. You'd never know by looking at her that a tumour was lurking in her lungs . . .

'Right, you pair – you ready for your lunch?' Expectant, they both looked up at me, trying to contain the food-induced excitement that only dogs can muster. 'That's a yes.' I laughed. I opened the Tupperware and handed them half a peanut-butter sandwich each.

Between the Crohn's and the worry, my appetite wasn't up to much, and I nibbled at a wrap as Maggie and Ri happily tucked into their sandwiches and chews. Discarding my barely touched lunch, I opened my flask and poured myself some tea.

Tears welling as I thought about tomorrow, I reached for Maggie's paw. Stroking her soft pads and the hairy bits between them with my thumb, I looked out across the sharp rocks to the desolate, empty expanse of cold, grey, seething water stretching off into the distance, reaching out towards the end of the world. It wasn't fair.

'Hey, lassies, fancy a film night? I think we might even have some ice cream.'

We were all tired from our long day in the fresh air, and back at home we sank blissfully into the soft pile of duvets I'd arranged in front of the wood burner. As the warmth from the fire lapped over us, Mags rested her chin on my knee and we tucked into our tub of salted caramel ice cream, her eyes following from spoon to tub and back again. I reached forward and pressed my face into her familiar warm fur, like I'd done a thousand times before, and wished I could pause time.

In the time since Mags' diagnosis, autumn had taken hold, and as day broke, the spectacular golds and browns of the Perthshire forests lit up our route south along the A9. Maggie was in the boot, making the most of the extra time in bed.

'You OK back there, toots?' I tried to add some cheer to my voice, but of course she could feel the dread and worry that had cloaked around me the last few weeks. I could sense the signs that my old pal panic was about to show its face, but Maggie really didn't need me to have a meltdown right now. I cranked up the stereo and, though it was the last thing I felt like doing, I tried to let music, singing and driving take the brunt of my emotions.

'Tea and toast, Mum?'

After her pre-op checks, we drove back to Kilmarnock to stay overnight with Mum and Dad. I knew I had to get some rest, but the chances of being able to sleep were slim to none. Tea and toast with yer mammy was made for times like this. As Maggie lay snoring in her bed by the radiator in the hallway, with her pal Peter – a black and white, very spoiled moggie – sound asleep, curled up between her paws, we drank our tea and blethered. Sometimes, we managed to distract ourselves for a while, but there was no escape and it was never long before we crashed back into the dreadful lurking reality. It was almost two a.m. by the time exhaustion got the better of us and we thought about trying to get some sleep.

We hugged each other goodnight in unspoken reassurance, and I went to brush my teeth. Mags and Peter were still lying wrapped around each other, snoring. I stopped and watched them for a few moments, Mags' eyes flickering and her paws taking her running somewhere in the dream world. I smiled and gave her a long kiss on the top of her head.

'I love you, Mags. I love you so, so much.'

I wanted to stay there forever, but instead I tucked a blanket round her shoulders and gave her one more kiss.

'Goodnight, sweetheart. I'll see you in the morning.'

'Here, eat this.' Mum handed me a roll.

'I don't want anything. I'm not hungry.'

'Eat it. You need to keep your strength up.'

We'd managed to get away early, to miss the Glasgow traffic, and we were making good time on our journey to the vet hospital. I knew I was doing the only thing I could, but this was hellish. I didn't want to do this to her, to put her through all this. I didn't want any of this to be happening. I glanced back at the boot, where Mags had gone to sleep, and I hoped that she was as blissfully unaware as she seemed. I felt as glad she didn't know what was coming as I felt guilty for not being able to tell her.

'Eat it,' fretted Mum. 'You need to keep strong for Mags.'

I took the roll and started to force it down, and she handed me a wee carton of orange juice.

'For the vitamin C,' she clucked.

'Come on, Mags, you must be needing a wee.'

The closer we'd got to the hospital, the more I'd wanted to turn the car round and flee, but we'd arrived, and had a few minutes to spare. As I fastened her lead, I gave her a big squeeze and kissed her soft, wrinkly forehead. As Maggie sniffed her way around the grass verge and young trees that dotted the well-kept lawn, we passed a couple of other folk doing the same as us, and I recognised the worry on the faces looking back at me. This happens every day, I thought. There was nothing special about our situation or our worry or our fear, but it didn't make it any less excruciatingly painful.

The reception of the hospital was bustling as another busy day got going. Mum and I took a seat on the plastic chairs in the waiting area, Maggie between us, taking in the scene, somehow managing to smile with her whole body, as usual. Even the immense suffocating dread weighing me down couldn't stop me smiling back at her. I loved her as much as it felt possible to love someone.

'Maggie Fleming? Hi, good morning. In you come.' A surgeon in blue scrubs was standing in the doorway of the consulting room, holding some paperwork.

Mum squeezed my hand.

'Right, Mags – that's us, darling. Come on, let's go.'

Cheerful as ever, Maggie trotted in and went off to introduce herself to the consultant and nurse. I could take Mags anywhere and, within seconds, she'd make new friends. I couldn't remember her ever making a fuss, causing any bother, doing anything other than being open and kind to everyone she met. I wanted to turn and run back to the car and put her in it and drive home. The thought of her being cut open was too much to bear.

Beside me, Mum was barely holding back her tears. I closed my eyes, took a deep breath and knelt down in front of Maggie. She looked at me, confused. Her ears were up, wrinkling her forehead, and her face was filled with worry. She knew something was up. I wrapped my arms around her and nestled into the ruff of her neck, smelling her warmth.

'Right, you – listen to me. I love you so much. So, so, so much. It's gaunnie be OK, you hear? I'm so sorry I have to do this. There was nothing else I could do, sweetheart. I'll see you soon. Please be OK. Please. I love you, Magpie.'

Crouching beside Mags, holding her tightly against me, I tried to take in as much as I could of what the surgeon was telling me about what was going to happen: when she'd go into theatre, when they'd call with news, what they were going to do, how long it would take . . .

Instead, I was thinking about our walks together. Loch Morlich, the Rothie walk, Lochindorb. Chasing sticks and paddling together in the Green Loch. The texts she sent when she was on her holidays with Mum and Dad, to let me know what adventures she had been getting up to that day. The times she'd spent lying beside me on the floor, for hours, unfed and unwalked, but never complaining, while my body and mind had writhed in inescapable agony. Gatecrashing picnics and making friends. Her smile. Playing 'chase me, chase me' with Ri. Lying together under a blanket. Sitting on her little mound in the garden, watching over her realm. Her night-night toast. Resting her chin on my leg. The velvety bump on her nose. The day we'd met . . .

'There's an inherent risk in any anaesthetic, and in any surgery.' The surgeon's voice brought me back to the reality I was trying desperately to escape.

Mags shifted uncomfortably in my arms. I was worrying her. 'Sorry, darling.'

'We need you to sign these forms to say that you understand the risks and you want to go ahead.'

I nodded. 'OK.' I stood up and inked my signature of love and betrayal on to the form.

As the door closed behind us, I turned and looked back through the glass pane. Maggie was being led out of the door on the opposite side of the room. She was searching for me, looking back over her shoulder to where I'd gone out, and for a moment our eyes met as the nurse gently coaxed her through the door, and then she was gone.

Back in Kilmarnock, Mum and I busied ourselves, keeping our minds distracted as best we could. I knew Mags would be in surgery by now. I wandered from bedroom to conservatory to living room, clutching my phone, and I tried to concentrate on some

Poundies admin. In the hallway, some kittens Mum had recently rescued from a building site were happily playing bat-the-ball and chasing each other up and down the stairs.

Mum appeared with a plate of beans on toast and a cup of tea, putting them on the coffee table in front of me, next to my phone.

'Eat,' she commanded.

'I'm not hun—'

'Eat.'

We'd been told to expect a call around two-ish. I felt like I was walking a thin line between two worlds. On one side, there was a safety net and a future; on the other, a drop into a futureless hell. Was Maggie still alive? Had she died and I didn't know? Surely I'd know if she had, somehow? Had they got the tumour out? Was she OK?

Just after half past two, my phone rang. My stomach lurched when I saw it was an Edinburgh number. This was it. I braced myself and answered.

'Uh-huh . . . Oh, thank you. Thank you so much . . .'

Maggie had made it through the surgery, and the vet was confident they'd got the tumour and good margins around it. She was groggy, but coming round, and she'd been strong all the way through. The surgeon had to go, but she'd call later to tell me more. For a few moments, I sat, bewildered, and played the conversation over in my head, to make sure I'd not imagined or dreamed it.

She was alive.

'Mum! Mum, where are you?'

Mum rushed through from the kitchen as I bolted down the stairs. She looked up at me, frantic, between hope and fear.

'She's through the surgery, Mum! She's through surgery. She's OK. Oh, thank fuck . . .' I crumpled to the floor, relief erupting out of me in sobs.

Maggie spent the next few days recuperating in the vet hospital. It had been a long, highly invasive procedure, and they'd had to remove part of her lung, as well as some of her oesophagus, where, unnoticed, the cancer had spread. She needed twenty-four-hour care and a lot of pain relief, and she'd also had a feeding peg put in, so she could be fed directly into her stomach, to give her oesophagus a chance to heal. The surgeon called me twice a day, keeping me up to date with how Mags was feeling and how her recovery was going. By the second day, she was going out for wees with the nurses, and by day three, they were having to coerce her back in, as she followed her nose from sniff to sniff. I asked if I could go in to see her, but they didn't allow visitors.

'The nurses all love her. She's very special.' The surgeon was getting very fond of Mags, and she knew how much I missed her and wanted to see her. She reassured me that she was getting plenty of love and affection, and that she'd be home soon. I desperately wanted to see her big, beaming smile and happy tail, her wrinkly forehead, and to wrap my arms around her and let her know everything was OK and that I had done all this to her because I loved her.

Four days after Maggie's surgery, on Saturday, it was the annual fundraising fair for Mum's charity, the Ayrshire branch of the Cat Action Trust 1977. Mum and a few helpers had spent hours planning and organising it – booking a hall, collecting tombola prizes from all over Kilmarnock, organising volunteers and paperwork. It was frantic chaos the night before, setting up the hall and ironing banners and hunting down Sellotape and Blu-Tack at three a.m. I was glad to be there to help; it was a good distraction.

There was a great turnout at the fair, and by the time we got back to Mum and Dad's that evening, we were exhausted. Mags' nurse had called just as we were leaving the hall, to give me an update. She was still doing well and everything was on track for her to come home the next day. We'd arranged to collect her at two p.m. I could finally accept that we'd fallen into the safety net and that our future together lay ahead. I didn't even try to contain my excitement; with the weight gone, I felt like I was floating.

Mum had disappeared up to the bedroom to fall asleep in front of *Casualty* for a while, and Dad was snoring away in the conservatory with an open book lying redundant across his chest. I decided to go for a lie down, too. It had been a tiring, worrying few weeks, and I could feel it taking its toll on my body. Up in my childhood bedroom, I wrapped an old candlewick blanket round my shoulders and cooried in. I loved being back at Mum and Dad's, especially in my old bedroom. Once home, always home. This time tomorrow, Maggie would be here, too. Glowing with happiness, I lay down and almost instantly fell asleep.

Groggy, I reached for my phone.

My mobile was ringing. An Edinburgh number. The vet hospital. *What time is it?* I wasn't due another update that night. *Fuck.*

'. . . There's nothing we can do . . . I'm so sorry . . .'

No. No. Please, no. This can't be happening.

Maggie had been given one last feed before her tube was due to be taken out for good. Somehow, it had accidentally slipped out of place, so, rather than the liquid going through the tube and into her stomach, it had flooded through her abdomen, coating her internal organs, causing what the surgeon told me was 'the worst case of peritonitis I've ever seen.' When the nurses found her, lying alone in her kennel, she had crashed in septic shock, heart racing and in agony. She'd been rushed to theatre, but it was hopeless. There was too much damage.

I pleaded to be able to see her, to be with her, saying I'd rush straight there.

There's no point, I was told. They couldn't let me in. It would be too late by the time I got there. There was nothing I could do.

'But I promised her . . .'

Just before eight p.m. on 24 October 2015, I gave my permission to end Maggie's life, and in that moment, a hundred miles away from me, Maggie died and the world I knew ended.

Frozen, I sat on the edge of the bed and looked at the floor, and, like a deep flesh wound that goes white before the blood comes, like the calm sea pulled back before the tsunami hits, for a few moments, I felt nothing.

Quietly, we got into the car. It was just past midday, and in two hours we'd be in Edinburgh, saying goodbye to Maggie's body – when we should have been picking her up to come home. Dad, stoic as always, was driving, and Mum sat in the back, sobbing and stunned by grief.

It was about half an hour into our journey, going down the hill just after the turn-off for Newton Mearns, when the aching, unmendable chasm opened up inside me. Thoughts circled in my mind – of my broken promise, of Maggie dying alone, of us never seeing each other again. I relived the last moment we saw each other, when our eyes met and we were pulled apart. I imagined the days Maggie had spent confused, wondering where I was and why I'd let this happen. A betrayal wrapped in love.

Maggie had died alone, but I had to cling on to the fact that she was carried through life by love. She knew love. She felt loved, and knowing that was the only thing that could even begin to break through this pain. I remembered the countless faces I'd seen looking out from dog pounds or factory farms, ill and dying, the lost, desperate, hopeless souls, broken spirits, tortured by loneliness. They'd never known love like Maggie had. They had truly died alone.

And, in that moment, a thought found me.

'The Maggie Fleming Animal Hospice.'

I turned to Dad and, briefly, our eyes met. I reached round to Mum. She gripped my hand and, through her grief, she smiled and nodded.

CHAPTER EIGHT

Osha Dosha Do, Osha Dosha Don't

'Osha! OSHA! Aye, you. Care to tell me why the contents of the bin are all over the hall? Never mind yer innocent face, I know it was you . . .'

A face full of bullmastiff cheek grinned up at me. Not a single damn was given. Big, bold, stubborn, loud, naughty, belligerent, ruled by her stomach and bone idle, Osha was a charming headache in dog form. Unquestioningly certain of her own magnificence, Osha believed that the world and everything in it was here to serve her, especially if she could eat it or sleep on it, or – savour the day – eat it while sleeping on it.

While Maggie had been going through her tests, I'd got a call about a middle-aged bullmastiff lass called Osha. Through Pounds for Poundies, Cathy and I had known each other for a while, and she'd heard about Osha from one of the pounds she helped. A few weeks before, Osha had been taken to the pound with a nasty, advanced and no-longer-treatable tumour on her anal gland. It was a long, upsetting story, but the gist of it was that Osha no longer had a family, so she was now living alone in a kennel, and she only had about six months to live. The ladies at the kennels who were looking after her really cared about Osha and wanted her to spend her last few months somewhere she could call home.

'I don't suppose you've got any room at the inn, Lexy? I can't think of anywhere else for her; everywhere is full . . .'

'I really don't, Cathy,' I said, trying to be practical, but already wondering if there was some way to make it work.

My health had improved and, with the pain mostly under control and my appetite back with a vengeance, I'd started to fill out and to look and feel more robust. I was doing things that, just a few months ago, I'd resigned myself to never being able to do again; I felt like I'd been rebooted.

Maggie, Ri, Annie and I were settled and content, and although, on the one hand, I didn't want to bring more stress to our lives and ruin the peace and equilibrium we'd found, on the other, I really wanted Osha to spend her last few months in a home with a family. Having a home and a friend to share their final days had mattered so much to George and Angus; I knew that it made such a difference to someone to be loved and to feel safe as they got ready to leave this place.

There would be logistical headaches and a difficult adjusting period, but I had a spare bedroom, plenty of time, and I'd made it work before, in a much more difficult situation. Once again, a decision made itself.

'I could throttle you, wummin!' I said.

'I thought you might say that!'

'Ha ha, aye, I know ye did! Right, let's get her transport sorted . . .'

A few days later, her chauffeur pulled into the drive, and out of the car swanned Osha. She was a big, solid lass, with a tan coat and brown eyes twinkling out from among the wrinkles. She looked exactly like the dog version of Grumpy Cat. Overflowing with self-confidence, she wasn't even slightly worried that she'd been bundled into a car in one place, driven a considerable distance, and bundled out of it in another place. She gave me a cursory sniff, emptied her bladder and set off, nose to the ground, to explore wherever she was.

It was instantly clear that Trouble had just landed.

'Osha. OSHA! Oi, gimme it. Gimme it. OSHA!'

Bit by bit, I extracted the soggy, half-chewed wrapper from her mouth, through her clenched teeth.

'Osha, that isnae edible. It's plastic. Ye cannae eat plastic.'

She looked at me like I'd missed the newsflash about the recent discovery of the amazing nutritional value of plastic.

'Let go, Osha. *Let go.*'

I was trying hard not to smile at her wee crooked front teeth that had all been given different instructions about which direction they were supposed to grow in. Finally, I won the battle of wills and, wiping the drool off my hands, I dropped the bits of wrapper back into the bin.

'Right, that's plenty out of you, today. I'm fed up with ye. Bed. On ye go. BED.'

She looked up at me, eyebrows raised. She had absolutely no intention of doing whatever that thing was that I just told her to do.

'Fine.'

Both of us knew there was only one way I was going to feel like I'd won this latest stand-off. I went to the cupboard to get one of her big chews and walked through to her bedroom. She swaggered in behind me and hauled herself up on to the double bed.

'Osha, ye'd sell yer soul for a sweetie in bed.'

She grinned at me.

'Aye, I know ye think yer funny. Here . . . enjoy.' I handed her the chew. 'I love you, Osha Dosha Do. Yer a pain in the arse.'

I rubbed my hand over her shoulders for a while as she chewed, and gave her a squeeze and a kiss on her wrinkly forehead.

'Night night, Osh.'

It was just as well I wasn't expecting a response.

I don't remember much from the weeks after Maggie died, but I was relieved that Osha settled quickly and painlessly. After all she'd been through, so long as Osha had a bed, a regular supply of food, a family and someone to give up their entire life to fulfil her every whim any time of night or day, she was happy. It was good for me to have the distraction of someone else to think about, and she was great fun to be around.

As the weeks went on, I worked on getting her and Ri to be pals, too. Ri was really clingy for a while, as she got used to the new ways of

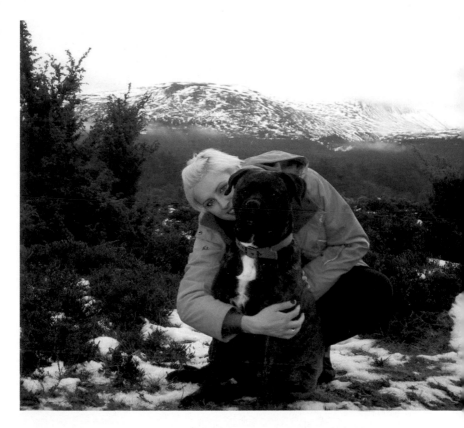

Above: Maggie and me in December 2010 on our 'Rothie' walk in the Cairngorms National Park near Aviemore with the haunting Lairig Gru pass in the background. © *Archie Fleming*

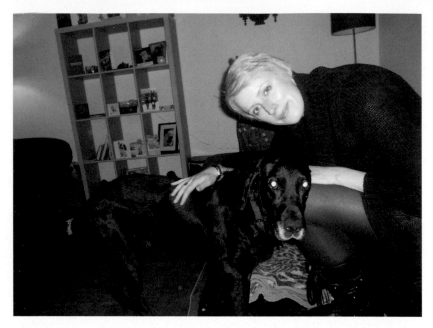

George not quite believing what was happening, but looking and feeling good and smelling a bit like coconuts after his wash and towel dry in our wee flat in Aviemore. 19th December 2010. © *Alexis Fleming*

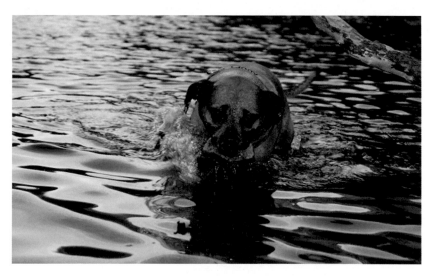

Annie on a mission, stone fishing in the River Druie near Aviemore circa summer 2013. This one was on the medium pile; not quite a king of stones, but a good one nonetheless. © *Alexis Fleming*

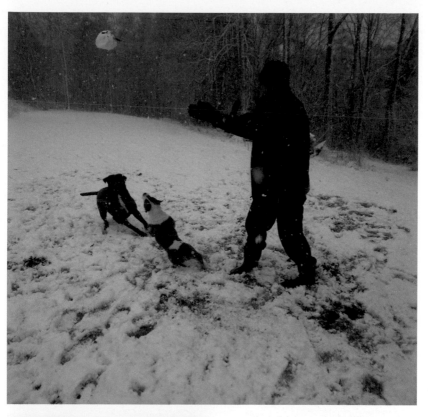

Above: Snowball fight! Maggie, Ri and Dad playing in the snow in the garden of our cottage in Ballindalloch in the winter of 2013/14. © *Alexis Fleming*

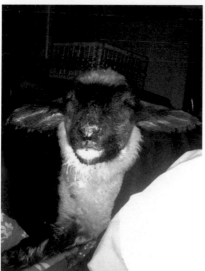

Left: Angus, sleepy and content after his bottle in front of the log burner, a few hours before he had to leave. September 2015. © *Alexis Fleming*

Right: Maggie taking a break from her morning perimeter sweep and enjoying the spring sunshine from her look-out spot in her garden at our cottage at Ballindalloch. April 2014.
© *Alexis Fleming*

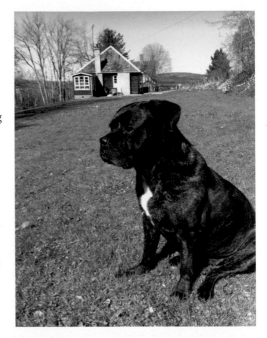

Below: Osha chasing smells in her favourite place, down in the wee bit of the world that time forgot. May 2016.
© *Alexis Fleming*

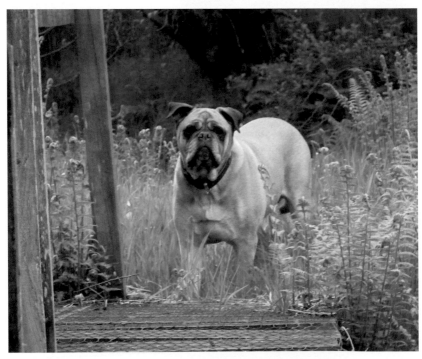

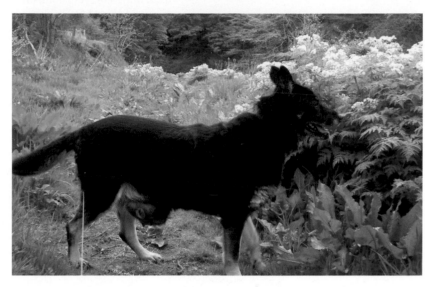

B's first walk after she arrived, and the tumour that threatened to end her life. In spite of everything, she was cheerful and loved hoovering up all the new smells after life in the city. May 2016. © *Alexis Fleming*

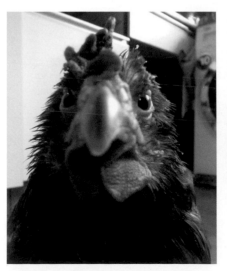

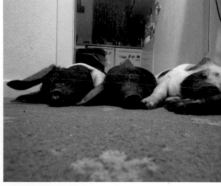

All tired out after another episode of Extreme Home Makeover. The delightful, exhausting chaos of December 2017. © *Alexis Fleming*

Georgia exploring the kitchen, wondering what to get up to next. July 2017. © *Alexis Fleming*

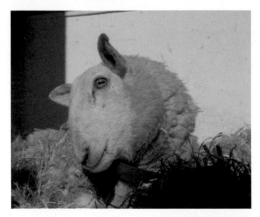

Left: Maya enjoying company, peace and sunshine as she took her final few steps in this life. February 2018.
© *Isa Rao*

Below: Gimli when I got out of hospital in June 2018, making sure I didn't pull another stunt like that again. 'I cannae bloody trust ye, wummin, off gallivanting without me . . .'
© *Archie Fleming*

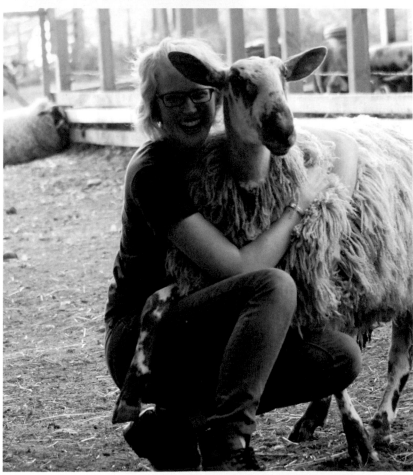

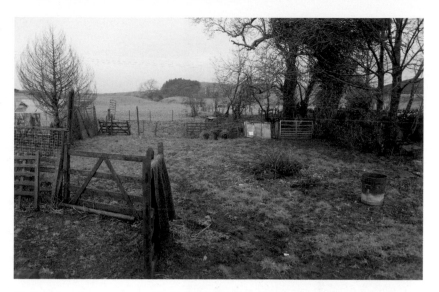

Definitely a doer-upper... My first view of Ringliggate in February 2018. Two years on, this wee bit of forgotten land has been transformed into a car park. © *Archie Fleming*

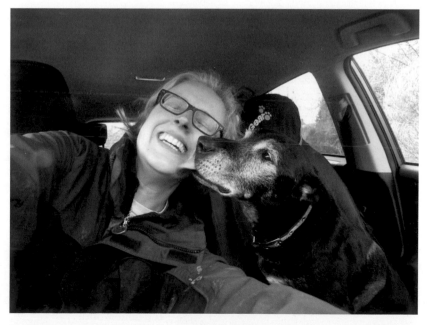

'WUMMIN! CAR! CHIPS! WUMMIN! WOOF! CAR! WUMMIN!' Bran and me in April 2017 on one of our many day trips in his CAR! © *Alexis Fleming*

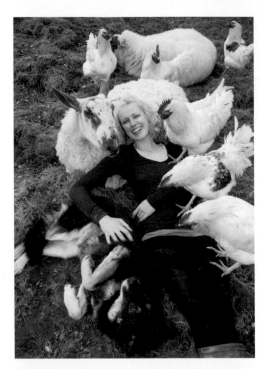

A Nice Place To Live. With
my family in our new home.
© *John Kirkby*

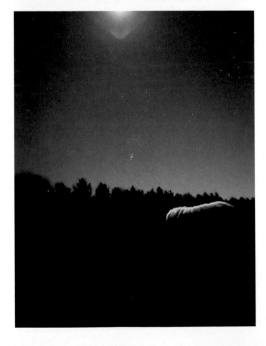

The same world,
with different highlights.
© *Kerry McCleary*

our changing family, but we were all finding our balance. There were a few minor disagreements, but I think Ri had the same inclination as me: it wasn't worth the bother. They'd learned to tolerate each other, and sometimes even dozed next to each other on the couch. But Osha liked her space and she sure as hell wasn't going to be a comfort blanket for an insecure, neurotic Staffie, while I think Ri felt a bit rejected by Osha's aloofness after her closeness with Maggie.

The tumour on Osha's anal gland was grim. It was large, about the size of a grapefruit, but if she noticed it, she didn't let on. We reckoned it had probably been growing for at least a couple of years; frustratingly, if something had been done when it first appeared, it would have been straightforward to take off and she wouldn't be in this situation. Now, because of where it was and its size, it wasn't feasible to remove it: there wouldn't be good enough margins to be sure of fully getting rid of it, so there would be a reasonable chance it would come back. It would also have been a 'dirty' surgery, with a brutal recovery and a high chance of the wound becoming infected. We'd seen a couple of vets and they both said the same thing: leave it alone.

Over time, as it grew, it would start to ulcerate and maybe even become necrotic as it reached tipping point and the skin and blood supply couldn't keep up with the rate at which it was growing. She'd had chest X-rays when she arrived, and there were signs of some spread to her lungs, and small, suspicious lumps were starting to appear on her mammary glands, too.

It was hard to accept, but, in terms of medical intervention, apart from giving her pain relief when she needed it, the best thing I could do for Osha was nothing at all. I could try to slow the growth of the tumours with good food and a happy, healthy life, and I could keep the skin supple with creams and supplements. But ultimately, one day soon, being alive would quickly be reduced to nothing but the endurance of pain for Osha. I didn't want her to go through that. I didn't want my friend's spirit to have to slowly fade away, trapped in her failing body. Osha was that twinkle looking out from the wrinkles; when that was gone, she was gone, whether her decaying body was still holding on or not. It hurt like hell, but ultimately there was only one way this was going to go, and it could either be really awful for her, or it could be really nice for her. I was dreading that moment coming, but there was nothing else I could do apart from be ready and prepared for it when it came – and, until it did, fit in as much food, sleep, naughtiness and adventure as we could. We might not get to decide whether we play the game or not, but that doesn't mean we can't tinker with the rules.

'Osh, look how many folk are following yer adventures. We should do ye a page.'

She was lying in a wood-burner-induced dwam in front of the stove. I'd been putting her stories on Facebook; it was nice to share how happy she was and what adventures she'd been having on her walks and days out to the beach or up to Elgin. I thought her own page would be good for her online pals, who liked to hear what nonsense she'd been up to.

'Aye, let's do that, Osha Dosha, plate washa. Let's get yer page made: Osha's Adventures. What d'ye think, Osh?'

Nothing. She was either sound asleep, or ignoring me.

Osha's favourite walk was down at the burn, a small stream flowing between damp, moss-covered rocks, which ran below an old humpback bridge and on down to the river below. She loved it there. She'd have followed the deer and pheasant smells in and out of the ferns all day if I didn't remind her that I existed and would like to go home at some point. As soon as I unhooked her, she'd trot off down the steps ahead of me and sway over the wooden bridge that was one heavy downpour away from becoming driftwood, straight into the muddy puddles on the other side.

It had been a few months since Maggie died. I'd really not been in the mood for Christmas; I never was, but even less so that year. By late January, around my birthday, I was feeling a bit more up to celebrating something, and Mum suggested I go down to stay with them for a few days. It was the first time I'd been to visit them without Mags, and although the car was full, it was painfully clear that someone was missing. Going to see her gran and gramps and her cousin Robbie for her holidays had been one of Mags' favourite things.

Robbie was a Staffie that Mum and Dad had adopted from a rescue around the same time that I'd got Annie and Ri. He'd had a chaotic start to life, and – combined with his innate Staffie neuroses and his own particular blend of hyperactivity and bonkersness – he'd spent his first six months at Mum and Dad's dialled up to twelve. Maggie had been really good for him, and her gentle go-with-the-flow energy had helped him calm his beans a bit. Now, he saved his hyperactive bonkersness for special occasions, like when his big cousin Osha came to stay.

'Nice new doors!' I shouted through to the kitchen as I opened the front door. Mum and Dad had been getting some work done on the house and, after an excruciating amount of deliberation and procrastination, they'd made a decision and had the doors fitted that week.

'Aye, finally. They're nice, though, aren't they?' Mum shouted back.

I wandered through to the kitchen to give her the obligatory bunch of flowers and packet of sweeties.

'Awww, they're lovely. They better have been reduced.' She laughed as we hugged hello.

'Yellow stickers all the way, Mum – as if I'd pay full price for yer flowers. Yer no' worth it.'

Smiling, Mum went to put the kettle on, while I went to unload the car and distribute Osha, Ri and our belongings to where they needed to be. We didn't know how Osha was with cats, so we had to be careful to keep her separate, and she'd been designated her sleeping quarters in my old bedroom upstairs. Once everyone was settled, I went through to the conservatory to see Annie.

A few months ago, Annie had gone to live with Mum and Dad permanently. I knew I'd let her down by bringing so many new dogs into the house, and Mum and Dad could give her the attention that she needed. I felt a lot of guilt about it and we missed each other, but I also knew how far we'd come together and how much our friendship had changed things for her. Mum, Dad and Annie were really fond of each other. My parents had turned their conservatory into her bedroom, and she was spending her retirement sniffing and sunning herself in the garden, digging holes in the grass and stone fishing down at the loch with Dad.

Late every night, Annie and Mum went on their 'school walkies', along the streets in the quiet housing estate where they lived and past the school where Mum used to teach. I got nightly texts from the pair of them to tell me about the smells that Annie had found during her forensic investigation of the grass verge, and how many times she'd wrapped her gran around a lamp post that night. When they got home, Mum covered her in kisses and then tucked her up on her couch with what I suspect was far too many blankets, hand-feeding her grand-dog her night-night toast. Annie had known and endured another way of living for a long time, and she deserved and relished every bit of the contentment and indulgence she'd finally found with my parents. She was totally spoiled and she loved it.

'Remember that time we lost Mags and Robbie in the park and eventually found them on the golf course, helping those golfers?' I said to Mum, as we wandered round the park with Osha.

'Aye, my Maggot-Pie was always such a good helper.' Mum smiled, her eyes red.

Grief still held hostage all the memories of the time we'd spent with Maggie, all the things that made us love her so much. The moments we'd had with her had been happy, but the space she'd left was still a raw, open wound.

As it went on, life would find ways to fill some of the cracks and chasms, but there were some broken pieces that, by their nature, could never be mended, and they'd always have sharp edges. Driving seemed to be when it hit me hardest, and there were times the grief would get hold of me so badly, I'd have to pull over and ride it out until it had exhausted itself.

It was delightful to see Osha so happy, with not a care in the world, and I loved that she was so content and enjoying her life so much. But I knew another bout in the ring with grief was on the horizon and getting closer by the day, and I didn't want to go through this fucking awful pain again. It was hard to know how to feel. Happiness and sorrow, presence and absence, laughter and tears, life and death: both sides of the same coin, existing at once, each as capable of justifying itself as the other.

At the other end of the leash, meanwhile, Osha was thinking of nothing but the possibility of finding something that was edible, or might once have been edible, or clearly had never been edible. Nose snuffling to the ground and slaver blowing in the wind, she was off in another world as Mum and I followed obediently behind her. Her nose gleefully led our slow bones up and down wee hills, through bushes and round trees. If she knew she had terminal cancer, it was barely an inconvenience to her. She only cared about what was under her nose or in her chops right this second. Osha was a lot of fun and a daily test of my patience.

*

Since the day I'd said goodbye to Maggie, I'd put the idea of the hospice to the back of my mind to let it idle for a while. I wanted to give myself a few months to think it through and consider it properly, and not make a decision when I was in the grip of grief. As the days passed and life began to reshape and refill around us, I started to give the idea of the hospice more thought.

Was I up to it physically, mentally and emotionally? How would I cope with so much death and grief? It would be a lot of responsibility, but that didn't really daunt me so much as whether I'd be able to do it justice, and whether I wanted to go through that pain even once more, never mind over and over again. Six months on, the grief that had hit me back in October often held me in as tight a grip as it ever had, and I genuinely wondered what was wrong with me that I was – for some reason – turning round and walking straight back towards the pain that I would do just about anything to get away from.

A few days into our visit, Mum and I had left Osha lying on the double bed in my old bedroom, absorbed in a peanut-butter-filled Kong, while we went out shopping. Normally, once Osha was in bed, Osha wasn't getting back out of bed for anything, especially if there was food in that bed, but normally there wasn't the opportunity for some cat-food prospecting across the frontier of the lovely new solid-oak door. She was sure she'd find treasure out there, if only she could find a way through . . .

'Awfurfuckssake, Osha! Wait till Dad sees this – we are gaunnie be in so much trouble. Osha, this is bad.'

I winced at the scratches gouged into Mum and Dad's lovely new oak door. They put up with so much. Ever since I could go out on my own, I'd been coming home with dogs I'd found wandering the streets – dogs that had caused some amount of bother, over the years. More than once, my parents had gone downstairs in the morning, after I'd been on a night out in Kilmarnock, and found a note on the dining-room door: *STOP! DOG!* I felt awful about their door, but I was skint and couldn't even offer to repair or replace it. Shame flushed up through me.

'Their new doors, Osha . . .'

She grinned at me.

'It's not funny.'

Five years later, you can still see the scratches and the holes from the sheet of plywood that Dad silently screwed on to protect his brand new, long-awaited, very expensive solid-oak door.

'Oh my God, Osha Dosha, yer gaunnie love this SO much!'

It was Osha's first adventure to a restaurant. We were making our way down the steep stairs into the Flying Duck, a basement bar in Glasgow city centre that served vegan burgers, hot dogs, mac cheese and loaded fries. It was my sort of food, and – being food – it was Osha's sort of food, too. We chose a table and settled in. Overwhelmed by choice, Mum, Dad and I sat in silence as we tried to make up our minds.

'Aw, shit, where is she?'

Without paying much attention, I'd tucked the loop of Osha's lead under my leg as I unbundled myself from my winter layers, and I'd got so absorbed in trying to convince myself that I'd be able to eat a macaroni-cheese burrito *and* a bowl of peanut butter and chilli jam fries that I'd forgotten I had a dog, and responsibilities other than mustering up some self-control and not ordering half the menu. I scanned the room. She couldn't go far, but she could definitely cause trouble. There was no sign of her.

I pushed my chair back and stood up to get a better look over towards the bar.

'Shit!'

Cursing my bag as I tripped over it, I rushed towards the kitchen.

'OSHA! Get oot of there!'

She was standing in the doorway of the kitchen, looking up at the chef, mesmerised. She'd found Eden. The source of all good things: The Place Where Food Came From.

I grabbed her harness and hauled her back.

'I'm so sorry,' I grovelled to the chef. 'She'd follow her stomach off a cliff, this one.'

He laughed, thankfully amused by the dog version of the Grumpy Cat standing looking at him like she'd just come face to face with the Creator. Back at the table, I put my chair leg through the loop of her lead.

'Yer a bloody liability, dug.'

She grinned at me.

When the food arrived, I got my camera ready to record her adventure for her Facebook pals, and put the red basket with her hot dog and fries down in front of her.

'Right, here ye are. Yer gaunnie love this. This is actually yer best day ever, isn't it? Ooooooo, here we go . . .'

In a few moments of utter bliss, she demolished the lot.

As spring started to slide in and shove winter to the side, the looming six-month mark that we had expected would bring an end to our time with Osha came and went. She was still looking and feeling great, and there were no signs yet of the tumour causing her any bother. It sometimes got a bit red, but she rarely acknowledged its existence. She could still do all the things she loved, and she was enjoying her adventures as much as ever.

'Right, Osha, bedtime. Out for a wee.'

She was draped apathetically over the couch, head hanging down off the side, going precisely nowhere.

'Osha. Oot. Now. NOW.'

Grudgingly, she began to peel herself off the couch. Deliberately taking her time going out the door, she paused and looked down. It dawned on me that I'd left a basket of eggs on the doorstep, and Osha 'Nostrils' Fleming had got wind of it. I made for the door to try to stop her, but she was off.

'Osha, no! Awfurfu— OSHA!'

In the light from the kitchen window, I could see her jogging up the garden, utterly delighted with herself, stringy raw egg dripping from her jowls.

'You are SO NAUGHTY!' I shouted up the garden.

I turned to go back inside.

'Don't be long,' I added, wasting my breath.

*

By March, I had mulled and procrastinated over the idea of the hospice for long enough. It was a terrifying leap into the unknown, but I needed to decide that I was going to commit to it. My battered old laptop and I were at it again as I started to build the foundations of the Maggie Fleming Animal Hospice. There were probably more reasons to talk myself out of it than there were reasons that convinced me it was a good idea, but regardless, the thought had taken hold.

Pounds for Poundies was still going strong. I'd just started a new side project called Consider a Staffie, and I'd had some nice T-shirts and other merchandise made for it. There were a few orders coming in, so I was going up to the post office in Aberlour quite often, and Osha liked to come with me. We'd walk up past the church, behind the shortbread factory, and circle back round through the woods. In the right places, I could let her off her lead, but she couldn't be entirely trusted, so I had to be on my toes.

It smelled great up there, especially if you had the nose of a bullmastiff, and I often watched the forklift trucks coming and going, and the gulls hovering overhead, waiting for a stray crumb, while Osha hoovered up the smells along the path.

'Oi! You – get back here.'

Osha had been swaggering ahead of me, weaving back and forth across the muddy path. Walking along behind her, I'd got distracted – away, chasing a thought.

Aw, shit.

'Osha. Osha! OSHA!'

There was no sign of her ahead of me on the path. I started

running; she could move, when she wanted to. Avoiding roots and puddles, I tried to see up into the woods. I couldn't see her between the trees, and she couldn't have got that far, surely?

Breathless, I stopped and looked around.

'Where the hell is she? Aw, no . . . no . . . nonononononono . . .'

I stared in horror down the hill. Osha was swaggering across the yard of the shortbread factory, heading straight for an open loading bay.

'The dog! Shit. THE DOG! WATCH OUT!'

Apart from the fact that she was effectively sauntering across the equivalent of a busy forklift A-road like she owned the place, Osha and her stomach roaming in a shortbread factory didn't bear thinking about. I threw myself down the tangled mess of the embankment as fast as I could.

'Osha! Stop!' I yelled, knowing as I shouted it that it was utterly pointless.

'Watch out . . . There's a dog!' I screamed, frantically trying to get someone's attention above the noise of the factory.

She'd stopped near the warehouse, nose to the air, checking she was still on course for Nirvana. With slightly more respect for health and safety than I'd just witnessed, I rushed across the yard towards her, breathless with exertion and panic, propelled by adrenaline.

'Stay there, Osha,' I said, as I approached her. 'DON'T MOVE.'

She grinned at me.

'D'ye think this is funny? Furfuckssake, Osha, ye just about got impaled on a forklift.' I clipped on her lead and then rubbed my temples with relief and exasperation. 'Honestly, dug, yer gaunnie be the end of me.'

Waving apologies to amused men in high-vis, we made our way back across the thoroughfare. Getting the idea that I really wasn't in the mood for any more fun and games, she didn't argue. Back up the embankment, still shaking, I bent down and wrapped my arms around her.

'Fucking hell, Osha. I take it something smelled good, aye?'

'Ye enjoying that, Dosha Do? Look at the state of ye.'

As spring and summer had come round, Osha had swapped sleeping in front of the wood burner for sleeping under the sun, and she was sprawled on the grass, completely indifferent to the existence of the chickens and turkeys dusting themselves near her. Over the last couple of weeks, she'd been slowing down, and although she was still enjoying her adventures, there had been a few times when I'd noticed her getting out of breath and finding it all a bit more strenuous than she used to, and I'd thought it best to cut our walk short and head back to the car.

On an afternoon in early June, the tumours in her lungs did what we always knew they would do and started to stake their claim on her. She'd been coughing a bit for a couple of days, and, as she hoisted herself up from her sun spot and plodded up the garden towards the cottage, a coughing fit seized her and started to rack her lungs. Head down, her ribs heaved with each cough, and every breath in wheezed and rattled. It was really hard to watch and must have been much harder for her to go through.

'Come on, darling, c'mere.'

I put my hand on her back and rubbed her shoulder blades. The tumour at her back end was getting noticeably bigger, and more angry too, and despite the ointments and creams, the skin was almost at its limit of being able to hold it all together.

'It's OK, Dosh. It's OK.'

I noticed a spot of blood on the grass.

There was no doubt left, and I had to accept that the moment had come. My stomach lurched.

Between coughs, she looked up at me, and for the first time, I saw fear in her eyes. I pulled her close.

'Aw, darling. It's gaunnie be OK, I promise. Come on, let's get ye inside.'

'Ye struggling, Osh?' I shifted over in bed to give her more room.

She was restless; though it was a still, clammy night, something so trivial didn't usually get between Osha and sleep. I leaned forward and dotted kisses on her head and face. She was upset and grouchy, not herself at all. I steadied myself, remembering why I'd wanted her to come and live with us in the first place.

'Oh, darling girl. It's too much now, eh? I know, darling. I know.'

Frustrated, she heaved herself up and turned around again to try to find some relief in another spot. Being able to sleep comfortably was a basic Osha requirement for life.

'I think maybe we'll call Ailidh in the morning, petal, see if we can go and see her? What do ye think?'

*

I stood quietly in the consulting room as Ailidh listened to Osha's chest and examined the tumour under her tail, and the ones that had sprung from nowhere on her belly. A bowl of gravy bones on the counter held Osh captivated – the promise of one, when the poking and prodding was over, enough to bribe her into still compliance for a few moments.

'Her lungs aren't sounding good.'

Ailidh stood up, clearly feeling the burden of what she had to tell me. She was fond of her patients and her compassion made difficult news easier to bear, but harder for her to give.

'It already sounds like there's a bit of fluid building up, and it's going to start making it harder for her to get comfortable when she's lying down. That tumour at the back is on the verge of ulcerating, too. I'd say she's uncomfortable, but I don't think she's sore yet.'

Snuffling and impatient, Osha edged closer to the counter.

'You've got a two-week window. If you do it in that time, she won't suffer. If you leave it any longer, she will.'

Ailidh was only confirming what I already knew, but I still felt like I'd been punched in the gut. In the same consulting room where George had taken his final steps a few years before, Mandi's words still hung in the air. *Better a week too early than an hour too late.*

As Osha ate her gravy bone, Ailidh prepared some medicines to make her more comfortable, and, held together by the resolve that, more than anything else, I didn't want my friend to suffer, we arranged that she'd come out to the cottage on Thursday and help Osha to die. I had two precious days left with my big girl.

*

'C'mon, let's go this way, Osha.' We wandered up the grass outside the row of shops and takeaways. She had a good sniff round a tree trunk, while I watched the world go by, holding back feelings that I'd prefer to let out at home.

'Aw, Osha . . . Guess what's back at the car? Doughnuts! You can eat what you want now, petal.'

Whatever I was talking about must have sounded like she was going to benefit from it somehow, so, obligingly, she trotted beside me back to the car to enjoy her naughty forbidden treat.

The things that made Osha Osha were starting to fade. She was cheerful and I still got a tail wag every now and then in reply to my fussing, but things she used to devour without even tasting couldn't tempt her appetite, and although she still tried, my heart sank each time she sniffed half-heartedly and turned away from something she used to love. With some encouragement, she still enjoyed scrambled egg and macaroni cheese and a few other things, and she could sometimes be tempted by a sweetie or two, but her trademark Osha appetite had gone.

I knelt on the floor in front of her and ran my hand across her head.

'Come on, ye can manage a wee bit more. You're Osha Dosha Do, of course ye can manage a bit more!'

She sniffed at the macaroni cheese and let me feed her a few mouthfuls.

'Ye've eaten about half – that's not a bad effort. Will we save the rest for later? I'll go and put it in the fridge. You stay here, darling. Get some rest.'

Weary, she looked at me. The medication Ailidh had given her was making her comfortable, but it was clear that she was getting fed up with her failing body, and she was starting to find this whole life thing a bit too much.

We woke up on Thursday to a beautiful June day. It was going to be a hot one. Osha had had a comfortable night, and we'd all had a good sleep. Ailidh was coming at around four o'clock, which gave me a few hours to make Osha's last day the best and most Osha day ever.

I looked over at her, sleeping on my bed, paws and eyes twitching, getting up to mischief somewhere in her dream world. She'd had much longer than we thought she would, and every moment of it had been good. She'd spent her days exactly how she wanted: eating, sleeping, doing things she wasn't supposed to and following her nose into new adventures. She had a huge bullmastiff heart and a sense of humour that made me laugh while tearing my hair out. Every night, on her way out for night-night wees, she'd check the doorstep, just in case the daft wummin had forgotten to lift the eggs again, and sometimes she struck gold, the thrill of finding forbidden treasure almost as good as the bounty itself.

Boldly, confidently, Osha had grabbed hold of life and enjoyed every moment. She didn't want to fade away. She didn't want that for herself any more than I wanted to see it happen to her. I didn't want to be looking her death in the face, and I didn't want her to leave. But, as much as it was the hardest thing in the world, it was also the easiest. The weight of the responsibility and power it gave me was grounding and sobering, but I had the chance to make a choice for her that would let her leave how she'd want to leave: with her dignity, doing the things she loved. It was the last thing I could do for my pal. It was part of the deal.

Without waking her, I tucked the blanket around her back, took a deep breath and went through to the kitchen to start the day.

'Osha, look at the state of ye!'

There was only one place to spend our walk together on this beautiful day: at our special place, down at the burn.

'Did you just face-plant in the mud, Osh?'

She grinned up at me, mud dripping off her eyebrows.

I shook my head. 'You're an idiot.' Laughing, we made our way up the hill to the car.

Back home, we got settled in the garden. We still had a couple of hours before Ailidh arrived.

'Hey, let's get some photos of us, Osh.' While I went to get the camera, Osha lay panting in the heat, smiling as I set up the camera for some family portraits.

'Osha Dosha Do, I love you, I love you so ve-ry much!' I sang to the Scooby Do tune.

Although she was a bit breathless and the coughing bouts still came every so often, she was cheerful and comfortable.

'Look at yer face.' I laughed. 'Yer lovin' it!'

After taking the photos, we shared a packet of M&S fruit chews, another once-forbidden bounty, and she was lost in chewy, sugary, sweetie bliss.

'Right, d'ye fancy some scrambled eggy?' I asked. 'I'll go and get it. Back soon.'

My stomach lurched as Ailidh's van pulled into the drive. I wanted to pause time. Under an impromptu sunshade made out of an old sheet, Osha was resting her chin on her paws, watching Ailidh and me make our way up the garden.

'We're definitely doing the right thing, aren't we? This is definitely the only thing we can do?'

I was desperate for reassurance that this final thing was the only thing left.

'Aye, it's the right thing, Lexy. Trust me. I've seen what happens when it's left too late. This is the best thing you can do for her. It will be really peaceful for her. It's a lot harder for you.'

On that warm June day, in her garden, after walks and photos and scrambled eggy and sweeties and love, Osha lay in the shade of her tent. As I stroked her lug and ran my other hand along her back, gently, kindly and with great care, Ailidh inserted the needle into Osha's leg.

As the sedative slowly took effect, I smiled through snot and tears and whispered to Osha about toast in bed, and face-planting in the mud, and raiding bins, and loitering in shortbread factories, and destroying doors, and macaroni cheese. I picked up the packet of sweeties. There were still a few left in the bag.

'Ye've got something left to do, Osh . . .'

And, in true Osha style, in a mess of slaver and ungraceful chomping and delight, she finished the last sweetie as she drifted to sleep.

Kneeling on the grass, I cradled her close, trying to let her know how much I loved her. I wanted that to be the last thing she felt, the thing she took with her to wherever she went next. She was leaving a good life, and I wanted it to be a good death that took her. Her breaths were deep, and slowing. My big, bold, naughty, funny girl was almost gone.

Wiping my nose on my sleeve, I leaned forward and whispered into her ear: 'Osha, ye know all those eggs ye pinched from the doorstep? I didnae leave them there by mistake . . .'

CHAPTER NINE

Flow

As life continued on and started to fill in the spaces that Osha had left, I kept myself busy building the hospice website and doing things to set in place the foundations. I was hesitant to take in any residents before I'd laid down deeper roots, and ideally not before I had built the actual hospice building itself. But that's not how life works.

Back in May, a couple of months after it had launched, the hospice welcomed its first official resident. Beryl – or 'B' as I called her – was a German shepherd/collie mix found wandering the streets of Salford, near Manchester, in desperate need of a good meal and a good brush, and with a weeping necrotic tumour the size of a rugby ball hanging from her belly.

She – and the tumour – had been neglected for a long time, probably years rather than months, and she was in a bad way. I knew the dog warden who picked her up, Erica, from the early days of Pounds for Poundies, and she'd been following and supporting the first tentative steps of the hospice over the last few weeks. Erica had taken B straight to the vet, and the news wasn't good. Given the size of the tumour and the likelihood that it had spread, the vet thought there wouldn't be anything to gain by removing it. At best, B had a couple of weeks before the pain became too much and there would be no choice but to end her life to spare her the suffering it was inevitably going to cause.

A couple of weeks of kindness and comfort was better than nothing at all, so Erica called to see if B could spend her final few days living with me. B needed somewhere to lay her hat *now*, not in a year's time, so at the end of May 2016, she came to stay.

B had long, thick black fur and a tail that could clear coffee tables in one sweep. She wore tan socks on each paw and her coordinating eyebrows rested above her soft, dark eyes. She was beautiful, but I could see she'd been through a lot. Worry and stress creased her brow, and her eyes were frantic and searching as she tried to put together the workings of her new world. I spent a lot of time with her in those first few days, reassuring her and helping her to find her feet. I knew she didn't have long, and I wanted it to be as calm and peaceful as it could be, but I felt like we were sitting on a ticking bomb as the display counted down the seconds. When I started the hospice, I'd expected to deal with death – of course I had – but I hadn't counted on facing it so soon.

I quickly realised that I was seeing signs that B was in pain. She was panting and licking at the tumour, and it was impossible for her to get comfortable with that awful open, weeping mass hanging menacingly beneath her. It was truly grim, one of the worst things I'd seen in a long time. I desperately wanted her to have as much time as possible being loved and comforted, but she couldn't go on like that. I was facing the first test of my resolve and responsibility, the first test of whether I had what it took to run an animal hospice. I called Ailidh and made an appointment to end my new friend's life. It felt so soon to have to go through all of this again, after Osha.

'Why don't we do some X-rays first?' suggested Ailidh. 'We've got nothing to lose.' I wanted to hold B close, but she wasn't much of a cuddler, so I kissed her head and stood up.

I certainly wasn't going to let any offer of hope go by. We still didn't know for sure that the cancer had spread. Going by the size of her tumour, everyone had assumed that it probably had, but what if it hadn't? What if it *could* be removed? It seemed so unlikely, but Ailidh was confident that, if there was no sign of spread in her lungs, there was a good chance she could get that God-awful thing off her.

B would have to be anaesthetised, regardless of what we chose to do, and once she was asleep, doing some X-rays wasn't going to cause her any extra stress or worry. If there was any chance B could keep living and enjoying life without pain, we had to take it. If there wasn't, if the cancer had spread, we'd end her life while she slept, and I would be just outside in the car, so I could be with her. Ailidh was right: we – and B – had nothing to lose.

'Let's do it.' Stuck in no-man's-land between desolation and hope, with no idea how to feel, I kissed B goodbye and handed her lead to Ailidh, and got ready for the agonising wait.

'I'll call you in about half an hour. Let's hope . . .'

Two weeks to live? Pah! B had other ideas.

The X-rays showed that, miraculously, there was no sign of the cancer having spread into her lungs. While B was asleep, Ailidh had managed to do a much better examination of the tumour, too. Although it looked awful, the mass wasn't actually rooted that deeply into her tissue. A biopsy didn't find any cancer cells, and though they were probably there, most of the lump seemed to be made up of inflammation and pus.

Five hours later, B staggered out of the surgery, groggy, sore, confused, but minus the tumour. It felt like our hospice had witnessed its first miracle.

I'd opened the floodgates. There was no going back now, and within a few weeks of B arriving, I'd welcomed another new pal to the hospice. And, boy, did everyone know about it.

'WUMMIN. WUMMIN! WOOF. WUMMIN!'

'Aye, Sir Branigan? Can I help ye?'

'WUMMIN! WOOF!'

'What d'ye want? D'ye want to go in the car, is that it? Right, OK, it's a nice day for it. Come on, then . . .'

Satisfied, Bran shoogled along behind me, wobbling on rickety, unsteady old legs, out of his bedroom and down the steps into the garden.

Bran was ancient, about eighteen years old, and he'd been found wandering the streets outside Edinburgh, alone, confused and half-blind, with untreated cancer on his spleen. He was picked up by the dog warden and taken to the pound to spend his mandatory seven days, but no one came for him. Given that there were a lot of young, healthy dogs in there who had slim to no chance of being rescued or adopted, there certainly wasn't a queue of folk waiting to adopt an anxiety-riddled, decrepit old dog with cancer. Bran was facing a bleak, lonely death.

In one of life's strange twists, Bran was found on his last day, by a rescue worker who was there to collect another dog. He was shouting frantically from behind the bars of his kennel, out of his mind with fear, and she couldn't bear to leave the old, sick, scared dog behind. Just in time, Bran had been thrown his lifeline.

At the rescue centre, he finally got the vet treatment he needed, and despite his age, he got through the major surgery to have the tumour removed, and his spleen with it. However, given his age and the deep-rooted anguish that incessantly shouted and whined and paced its way out of him, his vet thought that Brandon probably only had a few weeks left to live.

Sharon, the lady caring for him at the rescue, followed the new hospice page on Facebook, and in early June 2016, she sent me a link to a photo and a post desperately looking for a caring home where this poor old man could spend whatever time he had left in comfort. His Labrador-y face had once been focused and sharp, but now even his eyelashes had lost their colour, and his dark eyes looked out from behind grey curtains. But despite everything, behind those worried, frosted eyes, I could see that his spark still flickered on.

As usual, it would take a bit of juggling, but my instincts were telling me that, however long this sad auld dog had left, he and I were going to spend it together. And so, on a bright June day, Brandon shoogled his way into my life.

I soon realised that my ancient pal was held together with a huge heart, a formidable stamina and seventeen years of trauma and loneliness. Physically, he was healing almost miraculously well. He'd recovered from his surgery, and being spleen-less didn't seem to be causing him any issues. His short black fur started to take on a shine, and his wobbly step had a new spring in it. With some pain relief, supportive remedies, good food, gentle exercise and a pal by his side, the spark that had lurked behind his old eyes was spreading through him, and he was blossoming.

But the mental trauma cut deep. I didn't know what he'd endured in the years before we met, but I knew it wasn't love, security and kindness. For months, he frantically paced his bedroom, shouting at the walls, shouting at the ceiling, shouting at the door, shouting shouting shouting. On the bed, off the bed, clawing at the woodwork, trying to dig under his door. Desperate for love, but with no idea what to do with it when he got it, he lost his mind at the slightest hint of affection. He whined and shouted, panting and padding around on his tarpaulin-covered floor for hours until he exhausted himself. Anxiety, stress and never having cause to learn the rules for living in a home had left him woefully lacking in the toilet-training department, and every day there was a fresh unleashing of a tide of pee and poo all over his floor. It was a challenging and difficult few months for both of us, and I often struggled to keep my cool as the symptoms of his frantic anxiety – though completely understandable and forgivable – grated and frayed my nerves. Sharon had already warned me that he wouldn't tolerate other dogs, so, when it came to B, I had another Annie and Ri situation on my hands. The two had to be kept apart at all times – B slept in the sunroom, while Bran took over the spare bedroom. Meanwhile, Ri remained happily curled up in my bed.

As the months passed, Bran was going strong, stronger than ever, both physically and mentally. It had taken a while, but – as with most matters of the heart and soul – love, security, patience and time had done their thing, and Bran and I had found our rhythm. At last, he'd found his peace . . . and ruined everyone else's in the process.

'WOOF! CAR!!!!'

'Aye, I hear ye, I hear ye . . . Bloody hell, Bran. Hold yer horses!'

Bran had many charms, but grace, patience and volume control weren't among them.

Being about 146 years old, his voice was now his most powerful weapon and means of getting what he wanted, which was usually, quite simply, me. Strident, incessant and difficult to ignore at four a.m., Bran's MO was to shout his demands, wait five seconds, and, if the desired outcome hadn't been achieved in that time, shout them again more loudly, and repeat ad infinitum. At the slightest hint of light in his bedroom, he'd ping awake, ready to go; I'm pretty sure he was powered by photosynthesis. Winter had given a bit of respite, but as spring eased into a far-north-of-Scotland summer, I started to curse the almost-perpetual daylight. I tried blackout curtains, tiring him out before bedtime, ignoring him, not letting him nap during the day, calming diffusers, valerian, camomile tea, dancing naked round a cauldron, chanting incantations . . . but, nope – when Bran wanted something, he wasn't going to give up until he got it.

'Calm doon, dickhead. I hear ye. C'mere till I lift . . . Awfurfu— BRAN!'

Fed up of waiting, he launched himself forward and upwards, aiming for the boot of the car. His big clown paws scrambled at the edge as he tried to heave himself in, his back legs straining under his weight, only just holding him up. Half-in, half-out of the boot, he looked round at me, wondering what was taking me so long to fix the problem he'd created (again).

'Aw, I've to sort it, have I? How many times, Brandon? Ye cannae get in there by yersel.'

No matter how many times he tried and failed, and didn't even remotely embarrass himself, he was determined that neither I nor the basic laws of the universe were going to be right about this. I put my arm under his bum and heaved him up.

'CAR! WOOF! CAR! CAR!' he shouted merrily to anyone unfortunate enough to be within earshot, which I assumed would be pretty much everyone between us and Glasgow. As I turned the ignition and opened the windows, he padded his way around the boot, looking for the sweeties he knew would be hidden in his duvet.

'Ye getting them all, Shitter?'

It was the perfect mild, breezy day for a nap in his favourite place. I'd no idea why, but this auld dog just loved being in the car, even when it wasn't going anywhere.

'Right, I'm off to see to everybody else. It's not all aboot you, you know.'

Aye, it is.

'Aye, don't I bloody know it. C'mere and gie me a hug.' I kissed him and gave him a squeeze, while he ignored me and prospected for any remaining deposits of sweetie goldmines buried in the duvet.

Satisfied he'd found and devoured every last crumb, he turned to face me.

'I love ye, Branflake. Enjoy yer snooze.'

'Mornin', Gimli. How ye doing today, son? That some good grass?'

He looked up. 'MaaaaAAAA,' he shouted with his mouth full, and went back to his breakfast.

Bran and B had been with me for almost a year when my friend Lynn called to tell me about a disabled lamb who needed to find a new home or he would be shot. As a triplet, there simply hadn't been enough room for him and his siblings in their mum's womb. Squashed and squeezed in, Gim hadn't been put together quite right, and he'd been born with a twisted spine and displaced hip, which, although not painful, made it harder for him to get around, rendering him useless as a breeding ram.

When he first arrived at the hospice, Gimli could barely stand up, and I didn't have a lot of hope that he was going to make it. Then I discovered the problem: his tail had been docked, but because his deformity meant it curved back round and into his body, it hadn't been able to heal. It was infected deep into the bone, and for days, together with hefty daily injections of antibiotics and pain relief, he and I fought for his life. He was a strong, determined lad, though, even as a lamb, and he was far too keen to get up to nonsense to let something so trivial as a massive infection stop him. He eventually healed, and now he was standing without help and getting stronger and more mobile by the day. Longer term, I didn't know what the future held for Gimli as he got bigger and heavier, but for now he was a very content young lad.

Gimli and I hadn't known each other for long, but he'd already opened up a whole new world to me. I'd been around sheep my whole life, I was helping to bottle-feed lambs as soon as I could toddle, and I'd had those precious few days with Angus. But it wasn't until I met Gimli that I realised I'd never really got to know a sheep, not properly. And what a sheep he was.

One of my greatest discoveries was that Gimli was a great pillow. On warm days, we'd lie together on the grass and I'd prop my head up on the soft wool on his side, reading a book or dozing. He liked me to swing my legs around so he could rest his chin on them, and, like a sheep/human yin/yang, we'd lie, wrapped together, dozing in the sun. I'd never met anyone who could fall asleep so quickly and I'd try to stifle my laughter as he drifted off and started galloping through dream world, his eyes rolling and his nose twitching, his hooves going like the clappers. Some evenings, when summer gave us the best it had to offer, I'd take a sleeping bag out and we'd sleep together like that all night.

One of Gimli's greatest discoveries was Rich Tea biscuits. Since his first tentative taste, they'd become his crack. He was food obsessed in general, and it hadn't taken him long to learn how to open and rattle the letter box to get my attention – perhaps he was hoping it would become one of those magic Rich-Tea-dispensing letter boxes. He took any opportunity he could to break into the chicken shed, and I quickly realised I needed to have eyes in the back of my head if I had any hope of stopping him getting himself into trouble. Once, I found him wedged inside one of the wee chicken isolation coops. I've no idea how he managed to get in there, but I had to take it apart to get him out again.

Word about the hospice was spreading, and the local paper, the *Strathy*, had sent a photographer and journalist to do a piece on Bran and B, and my hopes and dreams for the hospice. It was the first media coverage we'd had, and I was delighted to see the faces of B and Bran beaming out of the paper.

'Look at you, Branflake. Yer famous . . . ish!'

Britt, a lovely lady who lived nearby, saw the article and very kindly offered to help. She was our first volunteer, and she came every Tuesday morning at half past ten to take Bran and B out for their walks.

The dogs looked forward to these walks with Britt, and I laughed as B did her arctic fox impression, jumping up and down on the spot and making a sound that was probably nearing the limits of human hearing. The excitement was too much to bear as the inept humans faffed about, putting on jackets and boots and all sorts of things you didn't need if you had a thick, glossy black coat to keep you warm.

'Calm yer jets, B! There's plenty time, doll!'

Bran and B each went separately, and Britt often took photos of them on their adventures in Aberlour or down along the Speyside Way, to share with their growing group of fans on Facebook. Afterwards, we always enjoyed a cup of tea and a blether, and I was grateful for her kindness and friendship.

It was a year and a half since Maggie had died, and smiles were coming easier and more often than tears, now, when I thought about her. Maggie had never known B, Bran and Gimli; my new pals and my old one would only ever meet through the pieces of herself that Maggie had left with me.

After she died, I tormented myself for months over whether or not I was capable enough to run an animal hospice. My grief for her was so raw, at the time, that I didn't know how I was going to cope with wave after wave of this anguish. But the idea wouldn't shift. I'd gone ahead and tentatively started the hospice on paper, still not sure I was up to it. But Bran and B couldn't wait for me to decide; they'd needed a friend whether I thought I was ready or not. I'd had no choice but to rip the armbands off and jump in, and now here we were, eighteen months later.

The basic, undeniable truth of it was that, because Maggie had died, my new friends had lived. And they hadn't just lived, they'd flourished. With the pieces of spirit that Maggie had left behind for us, old, neglected, dying souls had come alive. The wheel, always, must keep turning.

CHAPTER TEN

Georgia: Born with an Expiry Date

'Come on, everybody!' I called in a sing-song voice as I made my way up the garden carrying a bucket of mixed corn, a conga line of excited, bouncing hens following behind me. For a long time, I'd dreamed that one day I'd have some rescued hens clucking around, and that one of them was going to be called after my mum's mum, my granny Nessie, who'd died when I was twelve. A fiery Scottish redhead, with a wicked sense of humour and precisely no time for fools, I knew she'd have liked having a feisty red-feathered hen named after her. I had this idea in my head of being a tranquil, salt-of-the-earth chicken lady, sitting on a deckchair outside a wee chicken shed in my wellies, sipping a cup of steaming tea and reading a good book, while hens scratched and clucked around me and my best hen pal dozed on my knee. In my daydream, life with chickens was idyllic.

Not long after I moved to the cottage, by chance I heard about some hens desperately looking for homes to save them from the imminent horror of the slaughterhouse. Although I was still really unwell at the time, in every other way, the situation I'd dreamed of had come true: I had lots of interesting space for them to enjoy, and the time to care for them and provide them with a good life. Like a kid on Christmas morning, I called and offered some of them a home. I figured another reason to get out of bed in the morning would be good for me, too.

Two days later, after a very badly organised and almost disastrous handover in a supermarket car park, Nessie, Flora, Sadie, Janet, Margaret, Mary-Min, Shauna, Nettie, Clare, Karen, Jo and Kim cautiously stuck their heads out of their crate and, for the first time, saw that there was a world outside the metal factory walls. Gingerly, they stepped on to the grass and started to explore. For the first few days, they stayed close to the safety of their shed: inside was all they'd known. They startled easily and their bodies were pitifully scrawny and bald. For all they'd been through, though, I was amazed at how little time it took for the clucks and skips of excitement and the joy of freedom to start to replace the nervous jumps and cautious, mistrusting steps that were the understandable hallmarks of a lifetime of trauma.

As the days went by, good food, lots to do and the healing power of exploring in the wind and sun were bringing the lassies back to life. Their feathers were coming through and their once-anaemic, droopy combs had become perky and pink. It was a warm, dry summer, that year, and I spent a lot of time with them, getting to know their quirks and what they liked to get up to. Shouty Shauna liked to stand on one leg and shout about nothing, to no one. It was just a thing she did. Mary and Karen loved a cuddle, but some of them – including Nessie, who clearly didn't care much for my Granny-related nostalgia – were much more independent and didn't want much to do with me. They preferred to see what they could get up to down in the woods, or they'd take a saunter to the compost heap to see what the worm situation was up there.

On sunny days, I loved watching them as they earnestly dusted themselves in the dry mudbaths they'd dug, fluffing themselves up and turning on to one side, then the other, scratching and digging dust up on to their backs to keep bitey things at bay. They loved to stretch out and do a bit of sunbathing, eyes closed and wings fanned out, motionless, like they'd all just been mass-hypnotised by the sun. It always reminded me of the first time I'd ever seen chickens sunbathing, at Edgar's Mission. I'd run in a panic across the farm and burst into Pam's office to tell her that I didn't know what was happening, but all the chickens were dying at once. 'Pam, Pam, they've all keeled over . . . the chickens . . . I think they're all . . . having a stroke at the same time, or something . . .'

I'll never forget her face. 'They're sunbathing, you dickhead.'

'Hey, Margaret, what are ye up to today, darling? Here, fancy a bluebie?' I threw a few blueberries on the ground. 'Ha ha, look at ye. It's so exciting!'

They ran and bounced after the berries, running around, dodging and weaving, trying to avoid having the tasty treasure snatched out of their beaks, even though they'd just done exactly the same thing to someone else. Fairness didn't come into it; it was every hen for herself.

'Bloody hell, you lot, I wish I could get that excited about a blueberry. Right, who would like some . . . melon!' I threw half a watermelon on to the lawn and laughed as juicy, merry hell broke loose. 'Is that the most exciting thing that's ever happened, ladies?' I loved seeing them so happy, especially after all they'd been denied for so long. I settled down against a tree and opened my book. 'Oi, Mary, c'mere. I want a cuddle.' I picked up my best hen pal and popped her on to my knee. 'All I need is a cup of tea, eh, doll?'

'Buk buk,' she agreed, and snuggled in for a snooze.

When they first arrived, I didn't know much about chickens, so I launched myself into finding out all I could about how to care for them, what treats they liked and how to keep them happy and healthy. Surprisingly, one of the things that was really nutritious for them to eat was their own eggs. It sounded a bit cannibalistic but the shells were a good source of calcium for them, replacing what they lost with each egg they laid. They'd had a horrible life, so far, and I wanted to make life as good as it could be, now. There was so much to learn and it felt like, for everything I learned and got right, I'd get something else wrong or would have to improve or find another way. I suppose it was to be expected: it was a whole new world, and it was so different from anything I'd done before. What I hadn't anticipated, though, was that I'd have to learn so soon how to care for my new friends as they became ill. I'd read that wild chickens could live until they were about ten years old, and I'd assumed that once these eighteen-month-old hens had been saved from the factory, miraculously avoiding the slaughter-house, they'd have years of happy pottering ahead of them.

Flora was the first to become unwell. One morning, about three weeks after they arrived, I found her hunched over in the chicken shed, clearly feeling rotten. I'd no idea what was wrong, so I rushed her to the vet. The vet didn't have much experience of treating chickens, so Flora was given some painkillers and an antibiotic injection in the hope that it might help her, but other than that, I was at a loss as to what to do for her.

I took her indoors and wrapped her up in a blanket, and we sat on the sofa while I helped her to drink little bits of water with a syringe. I researched online and tried to find things I could do to help her, but she was fading so quickly that all I could do was watch helplessly as she got weaker and weaker in front of me. She'd only been out of the factory for three weeks; surely, she should have years to enjoy the freedom she'd only just found? She didn't seem to be sore, and I chatted to her quietly and tried to reassure her. Late one night, cuddled in beside me on the sofa, she took a few deep breaths and died. I didn't know if I'd done something wrong, or if I hadn't done enough, or if I'd missed something.

The more I researched and learned, the more I realised how naive I'd been. There was so much more going on in factory farming, other than the chickens just being locked up. Because they'd been genetically tinkered with to lay so many eggs – about ten times more than they should lay naturally – by the time they had laid the 350 eggs they were expected to during their year in the factory, often their bodies were worn out, diseased and falling apart. They were spent. Ovarian cancer, peritonitis, internal ruptures, egg-binding, infection – there was no shortage of things lurking and waiting to kill them. Flora, Nessie, Shauna – all of them had been born with a genetic burden that nothing could remedy. You could take the hens out of the factory, but you couldn't take the genetics out of the hen.

The next day, I dug a grave for Flora in the woods, as her sisters clucked and scratched around me, checking for worms. I cried and told her I was sorry – for what she'd been through, and for letting her down. As I marked where she lay with a little pile of stones, I was starting to realise that the reality of loving hens was not going to be anything like my naive, idyllic fantasy.

In the year that had passed since Osha left, the cannabis oil, plant medicine and a healthy diet had kept me well, for the most part. Although I still had some bad days, they were nowhere near the level of bad they'd been before. I had the energy to do all the things I wanted to do, and I even had energy left over to be enthusiastic about doing them. I still had cramps and discomfort, but apart from the occasional bad spell, it was bearable. I didn't dwell on it, but I sometimes thought about how close it had come.

When I was well, I loved life and its interesting, mysterious ways, and although my body had seemed determined to kill me, and I'd sometimes been tempted to bring the constant torment to an end once and for all myself, I'd never really wanted to die. Even now, it wasn't so much that I had almost died that bothered me, it was that I knew what I'd have missed out on if I had. I'd met George, Angus, Osha, Gimli, Bran and B, and my dream of having a few rescued chickens come and live with me had finally materialised, albeit not in exactly the way I'd expected. The hospice was putting down its roots, more people were finding out about it, and I was managing to raise enough money to keep it going and growing. It was still very early days, but it was coming together and I'd started to think about how it might develop in the future. There were still hard days, but I was grateful to be around to experience it all.

Making up for lost time, I started to find more things to get up to with my newfound energy. Getting to know the hen lassies and seeing their transformation – and learning about how the odds were stacked against them, even once they were free – had made me want to help more of them out of the factories and give them the chance to enjoy what freedom they could. I started volunteering to help out with the rescues, catching and crating the hens in the factories, and rehoming them from my cottage to folk in the area. I hated going into the factories. The stench of ammonia, the frantic noise, the bodies lying where they'd fallen: I could hardly bear it for an hour, never mind the thought of spending my life there. I couldn't get out fast enough, coughing and wheezing through the door and into the sunshine and air.

The factory I'd been to most recently, where Georgia had come from, had been particularly bad. It was the middle of summer, and inside the metal walls of the shed, the acrid ammonia, heat and dust caught the back of my throat and made me splutter and gag. As we chased, crawled, stretched, grabbed and shoved more than a thousand frantic, terrified hens into crates, it was obvious that there were a lot who were in a really bad way, and, by the look of it, probably didn't have long left to live. Now that I'd had some experience giving end-of-life care to hens, and with the hospice up and running, I offered to take the worst-affected birds home and fill however long they had left with all the good things they'd never known: peace and quiet, sunshine and fresh air, fresh grass and blueberries, and, when it came, a peaceful and dignified death. As the ten ladies and I drove home up the A9, all of us stinking and struggling to take it all in, I tried not to think about what was to come.

'Come on, darling girl, sup sup.' Wrapped in a blanket, Georgia was bleary-eyed as she unenthusiastically sipped her nutritional formula, drip by drip, from the syringe I was holding. Sitting up in my improvised bed on the living-room floor, leaning against the wall, I checked the time. It was just past three a.m.

Hilary and the other lassies were asleep in their carriers or in their wee beds next to me on the floor. Sharon, a traumatised lass who always had to be as close to me as she could be, was snoring peacefully. Her body was broken beyond repair and she was almost bald after a year of being bottom of the pecking order in a place where there was nowhere to escape the bullies who'd pecked and pulled at her. As egg after egg had taken its toll on a body not designed to lay so much, part of her intestinal tract had prolapsed, and the cannibalism and bacteria that followed had left her bloody and battling a vicious E. coli infection. The trauma of it all had got deep into her bones and she hated to be on her own; she desperately wanted the comfort of being close to someone all the time. As well as being tucked up close to me, she got a lot of comfort from the other hens. It was both lovely and heartbreaking to watch the gentleness of their friendship, as Georgia patiently let Sharon tuck her head under her wing and squeeze her body as close as she could as they snuggled up together in their crate.

Bran was in his spot next to me, sound asleep, his chin resting on his crossed paws. I took a deep breath, yawned, and tried to rub away the tiredness from my eyes. 'Come on, toots, try and take just a wee bit more . . .'

Georgia stretched her wing out behind her, balancing on one leg. 'Doing yer yoga, George?' I smiled and sat down beside her on the grass. It was early July and the weather was perfect for the ladies to get to know the world outside. 'Ye enjoying yourselves along there, lassies?' Some – like Hilary, a handful and a half of a hen, who had a horrible fungal crop infection, but was otherwise well – were stronger than others, and were up to a wee wander along the hedge to peck at the grass and bugs. But even the weaker ladies – like Sharon, who could only find the energy to lie on a blanket on the grass – were content just to be out in the fresh air and sun, watching the world go by, or napping, wrapped up cosy in their blankets.

I tried to make sure we got outside time every day. I'd carry everyone out, one by one, and give them their lunch – either a wee bowl of dried corn, fruit and scrambled or boiled egg, or a syringe of complete food, depending on what they were able to manage. Every day, I could see the weak lassies getting weaker, as their depleted, overworked bodies faltered and failed. It was heartbreaking, and there was nothing I could do to stop the ebb as my friends faded away from me. They wanted to live, but neither they nor I could turn back time or alter their genetics. Two lassies had already lost their fight. One after the other, in the wee hours of the morning, lying cuddled beside me in their beds, a few days into their freedom, they slipped away. Sometimes, it was all just too much for bodies and minds that had already been broken beyond repair. The damage had been done before I met them, and all I could do was make sure they were comfortable as their young lives faded away from them. I buried them in wee stone-marked graves in the woods, next to Flora.

It had been about two weeks since the rescue, and the long, worrying nights were blurring into long, frustrating days. All of the poorly lassies who'd come out of the factory needed intensive care. Some needed to be fed by syringe every couple of hours, day and night; some needed medication, or injections, or extra comfort as death crept closer. One by one, my friends were losing their fight, and already six had died. Some left really peacefully, in their own time, and, knowing what was coming, I'd taken a couple of lassies to the vet to hasten the inevitable and make it as peaceful and painless as it could be. One lassie, Tracy, had died a horrible, distressing death; a tumour I didn't know about had ruptured inside her, flooding her with toxins and contorting her neck backwards in spasms as she gasped and flapped her wings in awful convulsions. I had no idea what to do, except hold her and tell her over and over that I loved her and that she wasn't alone, until the spasms stopped and she lay limp on my knee, and I sat, shocked and weeping, on the living-room floor.

'Right, you, come on – eat the rest of yer breakfast.'

Georgia looked up at me.

'Look at the state of ye. There's more egg on yer face than in yer beak! C'mere and let me get a photo.' I lay belly-down on the linoleum and pointed the camera at her to get a hen's-eye view. She wobbled as fast as she could towards me. 'No' so close – yer all blurry, now!'

She loved looking at herself in the camera lens. Her head tilted to the side, giving her a permanently confused look, and the feathers on top of her head stuck up, adding a touch of the Ken Dodd. She looked like a cartoon chicken brought to life. I took a few blurry photos as she shoved her beak into the camera, and, bored now, she toddled off to find out what was down the side of the washing machine. She was into everything: if there was a nook or a cranny, Georgia was going to find out what was in it.

'Oi! You! Focus. Come here and eat yer breakfast, right this second, young lady!'

She turned and pottered back over to me, head tilted, feathers sticking up, little bits of scrambled egg in her eyebrows. I smiled at her as she wobbled towards me.

*

I knew Georgia and I were fighting a battle she wasn't going to win. One day soon, my pal was going to lose her fight, like her sisters had, and no matter how much she wanted to live, no matter how much I wanted her to live, I was going to have to hold her as she lost the battle. I tried to stay cheerful for her, for all of them, but I had to fight back tears as she toddled over to her little bowl of cut-up blueberries and strawberries, with a side of scrambled egg, and looked up at me, my little cartoon-chicken friend.

'Come on, darlin', you can manage some more. Ye need to keep yer strength up.'

She pecked at a blueberry and threw a bit of egg around for a few seconds.

'Come on, sweetheart, please, just a little bit more . . . please . . .' I held the wee bowl up under her beak, trying to give her a taste for it. 'Georgia, *come on*. Please. *Please*, just fucking eat!'

She startled and looked up at me, confused.

Shit. I closed my eyes and shame flushed my cheeks. 'Georgia, I'm so sorry . . .' I picked her up and cuddled her tight to my chest, sobbing into her feathers. 'I'm so sorry, darling. I'm so, so sorry. I didn't mean to scare ye. I'm so sorry.'

'Buk buk,' she reassured me, wriggling out of my arms to go and see what was down the side of the oven.

I crumpled to the floor as guilt and frustration welled up in hot tears and snot. I felt like I'd been hollowed out. With the last drop of energy I had, I stood up and left Georgia not eating her breakfast in the kitchen, went through to the bathroom, locked the door, fell to the floor and screamed.

Guilt tore at me for all the times I'd messed up and missed someone's lunchtime, or not known about a tumour, or lost my temper and shamed myself and upset everyone around me with a frustrated tantrum. Bran was as demanding as ever, shouting incessantly all day and all night for his every need to be met instantly, and it took a fair bit of time to care for the other chicken folk outside and to do the hospice admin. I had help with the dog walking, but it was stressful in the cottage, as I tripped over crates and chickens and dollops of chicken shit. Stress tied my guts in knots and it was hard to breathe through the tenseness in my chest. Crohn's thrives on stress, and a creeping fatigue and gnawing ache in my right-hand side was starting to rear its head. I'd always tended towards comfort starving rather than comfort eating, and I was surviving on the few crisps and hummus I shoved in my face every now and then, when I remembered and had time. My bed was made of folded-over duvets on the living-room floor; it was comfy enough, but I was snatching naps with one ear open, constantly listening in case anyone needed anything. One after the other, I was watching my pals lose their fight, young lassies who should have had years ahead of them, who, no matter what I did and no matter how much they wanted to live, were going to die.

It had been about three weeks since they left the factory, and all but two of the hens had lost their fight. I'd decided to get post-mortem exams done to find out exactly how they'd died, what horrible disease or decay had ended their lives. I had no idea, so I guessed that many other folk would have no idea, either, and I thought, if I could show people what had happened to them and why, then I could at least make their deaths mean something.

'Hilary, stop eating the paint off the skirting boards, please. HILARY! Right, that's it, outside. On ye go . . .'

Hilary was still going strong and causing as much bother as she possibly could. I'd never met a hen with such a sense of humour, who could get up to so much nonsense. She lived in the house, refusing to go outside to live with the others, and I'd often walk into the kitchen and find her standing on top of the bread maker, or – once – inside the soup pot, with the dogs' fresh home-made dinner in it, helping herself. She was a hen and a half.

But while Hilary caused all sorts of merry mischief, Georgia was fading. Her spirit was hanging on, but all the good food, fresh air, sunshine and love in the world wasn't going to fix the diseased and depleted body that carried it.

'Let's go outside, toots, hey? Go and get some fresh air?'

Georgia was in her favourite place: wrapped in a wee blanket, cuddled into my chest.

I leaned forward and kissed her head. 'I love you, darling girl.'

Hearing my voice, she roused and looked at me with a tired amber eye.

I smiled. She was so delicate in so many ways, but so strong in so many others. 'Yer so pretty, Georgie.' I kissed her beak and tucked the blanket around her. 'We've got to stay all cosy. Right, let's go and see what's going on outside, eh? Will that be nice?'

We walked around the garden together for a while, Georgia tucked cosily inside my fleece, swallows swooping and dancing around us. The stones in the drive crunched under my feet as we wandered around, seeing what everyone was up to, Bran shoogling along behind us. Her eyes were closed and I wasn't sure how much she was taking in, but I blethered away to her.

'Oh, hey, darling, look – we've got a new caravan! Let's go and see what's in there.'

Even a few days ago, she'd have been so excited to wobble her way around this fascinating new place and investigate all its mysterious nooks and crannies.

'Look, what's in here?' I opened cupboards and showed her all the places she'd have explored, if she'd been able. I closed my eyes and held her in close. Things being different, she'd have loved this adventure. 'Not today, though, eh, darling? Not today . . .'

Outside, the sun was high in the sky and warm on our faces. We sat on the grass in front of the cottage and Bran settled himself down beside us. A cuckoo was calling from across the valley.

'Aw, sweetheart, you're so tired.'

Her breathing was slow and getting slower, and her eyes flickered, seeing things I'd never know.

'Remember the bluebies, Georgie? Ye always had food all over yer face.' I smiled, thinking about the state she used to get into, eating her dinner. 'And remember that time you couldn't work out how to get out from behind the door?'

In our three weeks together, my wee red-feathered cartoon-chicken friend and I had explored the world, enjoying its tasty fruity treats and its warm sun and nooks and crannies. Although it had been for such a painfully short time, she had known the good things, the things that made life worth living. It was a world she might never have known existed and she might never have known those things. What a blessing those days were.

I couldn't change what had gone before. Georgia had been born with an expiry date. She'd been born to die, one way or another: alone and afraid, having never really lived; or safe and loved, and free. Her final tiredness was here, now, and wrapped up close inside my fleece, like she loved so much, my friend was slipping away. We might not always be able to stop death, but I was starting to work out that maybe there could be peace and dignity amongst the sorrow.

CHAPTER ELEVEN

Crannog

'I'm bloody knackered, Brandon. D'ye care?'

Sprawled in a contented stupor in front of the wood burner, he didn't even do me the courtesy of opening an eye and pretending to be interested.

Nope.

'Naw, didn't think so.'

I fell on to the sofa, sweaty and stinking of pigs. I had reached that eerily calm, slightly delirious place – way past the exhaustion and tears, and down the slippery slope towards maniacal laughter. I didn't actually know how it was possible to be this tired. Four-piglets-living-in-the-kitchen tired was a whole new experience of exhaustion.

I'd lost track of the days, but it was past Christmas, and Hogmanay was still to come. It didn't really matter what day it was anymore, though; every day was pretty much the same blur of walking, filling food buckets, cleaning chicken poo from sheds, driving somewhere for a walk, and answering Bran's every 'WOOF! WUMMIN!' whim. There was a lot of boring, necessary admin, and I was always worried about how to pay for food, bedding and vet bills – and everything else – and, as more animals joined my family, there was almost always someone who needed intensive care. It was usually a hen lassie whose past life and biology was starting to outpace her will to live, and it was often a losing battle. It seemed endless at times, and tiredness and anxiety had seeped into my bones. Supervising and doing as good a job as I could of cleaning up after the unfathomable chaos of four giddily rampaging piglets' worth of destruction took about six hours a day, but I could have sworn I was doing it from the second I got up till the second I fell, knackered and stinking, in a mess on the couch, usually well past midnight.

Around mid-November, my friend Hannah had found out about the piglet boys from someone she'd met locally who was fattening them up to be killed for Christmas. Knowing what that would mean for them, she wanted to try to help them, but she lived in the suburbs of Aberdeen and had nowhere for them to live. Sanctuaries are never short of requests to take pigs, and our desperate plea for these four lads was just another of many that week. We were getting nowhere. I already had two pigs, Charlotte and Emily, who were a rare kunekune breed from New Zealand and had been in need of a new home. They'd come to stay at the start of the year, and what had been Maggie's beautiful garden, which she'd been so proud of, had become an embarrassing and increasingly unliveable mudbath. Dad and I had built a small wooden fenced area for them, which contained the mud a bit, but there was no way it could take another four sets of snouts and trotters.

We were still trying to find somewhere for them to go when Hannah called one morning, frantic, to say that one of them – the smallest, weakest guy – was going to be killed later that day because he had a hernia. Although it was harmless, it made him unlikely to sell for the right price, so he had to go. It was a life or death decision moment; there was nowhere else for them to go, and the only option that would save them was for me to foster them until we could find a permanent home. It was too cold for them to be outside in a pig arc without their mum, and the two small gardening sheds were now homes for the turkeys and chickens. The only safe space I had for them was my kitchen. It was clearly inappropriate, and even the thought of it made me want to run away, but it was the only space I had and it was that or death for them. I got out the biggest dog crate I had, ordered a few bags of pig food, lifted a few things that were likely to get knocked over out of the way, and thought I was prepared.

The boys were about seven weeks old and were each about the size of a Jack Russell when I met them. The night that Hannah dropped them off, after the novelty and hilarity of *Holy hell, there are four piglets in the kitchen!* had worn off, I knelt beside their crate in the wee small hours and watched Andrew, Carl, Barnaby and the littlest lad with the hernia, whom I called Brian Baby, fall asleep.

I watched them for about an hour, a pile of piglets snoring and murmuring in their sleep as they twitched their beautiful, perfect snouts and wriggled. They had snuggled in so close together that it was actually impossible to tell which trotter, curly tail or snout belonged to whom. When one moved and a trotter got shoved into a delicate bit, they'd squeal, moan, protest, groan, grunt, rearrange themselves, and instantly fall back to sleep again. Sitting watching them there, in the dimly lit kitchen, I'd fallen in love.

The power of a mammy's love got me through a lot, those first few weeks. I knew before they arrived that it would be hard work having four piglets living in the kitchen, but – bloody hell – it turns out that I'd had no idea what hard work was before Andrew, Carl, Barnaby and Brian, and their ridiculously strong snouts and willpower to match, bulldozed their way into my life.

'Awfurfuckssake, Barnaby, get out of the fridge!'

Barnaby was the smart guy of the bunch, who always worked out how to break into, knock over or destroy things first, and then taught his brothers how to join in. Since he'd first discovered that the kitchen cupboard doors opened – breaking into the veg supply and running off, delightedly munching an onion – he'd made it his prime purpose to open all of the cupboard doors in the kitchen, every day, and empty the contents all over the cottage. I held the cupboard doors closed with every limb – right hand on fridge, left leg stretched to full capacity in an attempt to fortify the cupboard under the sink, like I was playing some sort of weird, piglet edition of Twister – but he was a smart and fast adversary.

'Aw, Barnaby . . . Nooo!' As I was putting the bottles of cleaning stuff back into the cupboard he'd just removed them from, he seized his chance and made for the holy grail: the fridge. With the help of his entourage, he'd emptied everything on to the floor in an instant, knocked all the shelves down, trampled it all under-trotter, and he was now channelling his inner Jackson Pollock all over the walls and floor with a carton of Alpro custard.

'Ooof oof oof!'

'Andrew . . . No, son . . . Not now . . . Oh, bloody hell . . .'

Andrew, meanwhile, was the instigator of playtime; when he fancied a game of zoomies up and down the hall, he'd *ooof-ooof-ooof*, getting louder and faster, winding his brothers up until they were in the mood for the same daftness. Every morning and evening, they'd spend two hours playing at zoomies, throwing around the dogs' toys I'd given them in the futile hope that it would stop them eating more holes in the walls, chasing each other and hurdling a chest of drawers they'd upended, and delightedly scratching their butts on the door frames and the vacuum cleaner. While the other boys drank, Andy liked to blow bubbles in his water bowl, sending water up and over the sides, and 'Collapsey Carl' loved to throw himself across my knee and have his belly scratched, no matter that he was now closer to the size of a Great Dane than a Jack Russell. I'm pretty certain that Brian Baby had precisely no idea what was going on most of the time, but it didn't seem to worry him much.

Clearing up the devastation they caused during their playtimes each day took hours, and as soon as I started to see the signs that they had tired themselves out, I'd get on with cleaning walls and floors – scrubbing, mopping and putting everything back together again. It was relentless; I'd just be finishing when they'd wake up, ready to start the whole thing over again. Impractical, stressful and exhausting as it was, though, the chaos and disruption and the holes in walls were a small and temporary price to pay in the grand scheme of things, if it meant the boys were safe and had their whole lives ahead of them. I was aware that a lot of folk would have – quite sensibly – drawn the line way before inviting piglets into their kitchen, but necessity and a willingness to try most things, if it meant someone didn't have to go through what the boys would have gone through, had left me line-less, and with a cottage full of piglets.

Every night ended much the same: I'd be desperate to be clean and in bed, but the shower and my bed were all the way in the next room. Bran was sound asleep in front of the fire; he wasn't going anywhere. No one but Bran was around to smell me, and his nose worked about as well as his eyes and lugs. I could hear the boys snoring from their crate next door, four snouts lined up, all tired out from their *Extreme Makeover: Home Edition* adventures. *Fuck it.* I pulled the throw covering the couch around me, knowing I would regret it when I woke up at four a.m. with a crick in my neck and wishing I'd been sensible, but I was too tired to care.

'Lexybee! We did it! We've been chosen!'

'Yer kidding, Isa . . . What, seriously? We're gaunnie make the film, for real?'

A few months before, through mutual interests and under the

guiding hand of being in the right place at the right time, my path had crossed Isa's early on a beautiful August morning, as we unfolded ourselves from our respective tents into an overgrown field, just outside Aberdeen. I was on a Hunt Saboteurs training weekend, learning how to use non-violent action to disrupt hunts. Isa was a neuroscientist and budding documentary maker, and as we sat cross-legged, breakfasting on warm hummus and stale bread, we got blethering about our work, lives and hopes. That night, we talked and laughed around the campfire, while I told stories about Osha, Gimli, Bran, B and all the other folk who lived at the hospice. At the end of the weekend, we swapped numbers and said we'd keep in touch.

Around mid-October, Isa called to tell me about a competition she'd heard of that was being organised by the Scottish Documentary Institute. Three winning documentary pitches would be chosen to be made into fifteen-minute shorts, with full support and funding from the Institute and a premiere at the prestigious Edinburgh International Film Festival. It was open to new documentary makers, and that year's theme was 'Love'.

'It's perfect, Lex. We can show the love between you and the animals at the hospice, the relationship you have with them. Especially the sheep . . .'

Since Gimli had *MaaaaAAAAA*ed his way into my life and heart, I'd fallen in love with sheep – head over heels, completely besotted. The Big Woolly Bastard and his friendship and love had changed a lot for me, and I was fired up about showing other people what I'd found: that there was so much more to sheep than standing in fields and eating grass. Although Isa and I knew there would be hundreds of entries, and the thought of being the subject of a film and having a camera crew following me around was the perfect fuel for my anxiety, the opportunity to potentially change hearts and minds about sheep, and other animals that folk rarely thought about, was too good not to at least give it a shot.

I recorded a shaky video, on an old SLR, of me and Gimli sitting together in the garden, Gim headbutting into me while I massaged his neck and nervously muttered something about what great friends sheep are and how much I love them.

'See you, Gim? You're gaunnie change how folk see sheep. Y'hear me?' Together, we had a job to do.

Isa did all the actual work on the application, and a few days later, we submitted our entry.

The weeks went on in the blur of daily tasks, and, being my usual Little Miss Pessimistic self, I'd already written the film off in my head. I didn't think there was really any hope that a short documentary about friendship, love and sheep had a chance.

So, when Isa called to tell me that our pitch had got through to a shortlist of twelve, I was astonished. For the next round, we had to make a three-minute short, filmed at the cottage. We arranged that Isa would come up to stay, and over a few bitterly cold, dreich late-November days, we worked on our few minutes of footage. Then, we waited.

Now, weeks later, Isa was telling me that our film had been chosen out of all films entered in the competition, and I could hardly believe it. 'For real, Isa, we won? We actually won?!'

'For real, Lex. We're making a film!'

The words were so unlikely that I felt like I was already in a movie. It was the day before my birthday, three years to the day since I'd been given six weeks to live. I was delighted, but overwhelmed; so much had changed in those years. Back then, I wouldn't have recognised myself now. I'd fought for my life and won, but I hadn't been able to save Maggie's. I'd battled, dug deep, wobbled, fallen, picked myself up, succeeded in some things and failed in others. I'd fallen in love many times, and had held the friends I loved as they died. My dream of starting the hospice in Maggie's name had come to life, and the ripples I'd always hoped it would create were starting to spread out across my wee bit of the world – and now possibly further. So much was happening, and the hows and whys were still a mystery to me. It was exciting, and it was what I'd hoped for, but the lack-of-confidence gremlin and the too-good-to-be-true fear were never far from my back.

'I don't think I can do this, Mum. I cannae be in front of a camera . . . I don't know how . . . Why would anyone want to watch a film about how much I love sheep? It's stupid to think anyone wants to hear it. I'm gaunnie have to tell Isa I cannae do it.'

Mum recognised the signs of the emotional mess that was brewing. 'It's going to be fine. Look, just accept it. They wouldn't have chosen it if they didn't want to know more.'

I searched my mind for inner reassurance. *You can't do this. There's no way you can do this.*

'Relax,' Mum soothed. 'It's gaunnie be fine.'

*

The piglets were finally big enough to be outside, which had solved one problem, but created another. The small piece of land Dad and I had prepared for them, digging and levelling slabs into the frozen mud as the snow fluttered around us, had turned into a mudbath within a couple of days of their snouts getting to work on it. The cottage was a disaster zone: there were holes in the kitchen walls and bits of the linoleum were missing, presumed chewed, and although I'd gone through gallons of disinfectants and cleaners over the last two months, the carpet in the hallway still smelled like a pig urinal. I was trying, but it was an embarrassing chaos, and I was ashamed for it to be filmed for the world to see. Dad and I had spent a few days tidying the place up before Isa and the crew arrived, but with too many animals in too small an area, there was only so much we could fix.

Against the cold, leafless, lifeless backdrop of February 2018, we started filming. Isa had brought in two folk to help: Adelaida, as director of photography, and Scott, as the sound engineer. Hilary, the boldest chicken in the west and ever the flirt, instantly fell in love with Scott, and temporarily abandoned Operation: Remove Wallpaper to spend her days standing at his feet, looking up at him adoringly, while he spent his days trying to do his job and not trip over his one-chicken fan club. Although the setting made me cringe, it was easy to capture the love that kept the whole thing together. Isa was a natural as director, and, in a Shyamalan-worthy plot twist, I discovered that I absolutely loved being in front of a camera. So did Bran, my old dog shadow, who shoogled along behind me in his wee blue winter fleece, hoovering up chicken shit as he went and insisting on being in every shot.

'I want an award for this, Isa; Best Laundry Folding 2018.'

'For sure, Lexybee. The award is already yours!'

I sat on my bed in the dim lamplight, folding my clothes, doubling over in pain. The Crohn's was rearing its ugly head again, and the bit of intestine that had been so badly damaged before was starting to cause problems. It felt like it was getting more inflamed, and the early signs of blockages were making themselves known: cramps, nausea, vomiting and exhaustion. The incessant tiredness wasn't just from the never-ending tasks each day; I could feel my body starting to fail again, but I had so much to do that I couldn't stop and rest. I was worried: I really didn't want to go back to that life, if I could even call it that, and now I had a lot more to lose than before. In the documentary, we wanted to show the effects the disease had on me, and nothing was more everyday normal than folding laundry, doubled over in pain.

A few days into filming, I got a call from someone asking if I could take a poorly sheep. She'd been living alone in a barn for a few weeks, barely able to walk, suffering from what sounded like a brain trauma or disease. She needed end-of-life care, and the timing of it was astonishing; her story would be captured in our film about love, sheep and overcoming life's hurdles.

It was clear, when I met her for the handover in a lay-by, that she was in a really bad way. Half of her fleece was gone from one side and her skin was covered in scabs. Her eye on the same side was badly damaged from the hay that had been poking into it as she lay prostrate on her side, unable to get up. She'd been alone for six weeks, with one visit a day for food, lying on concrete in northern Scotland's deep winter freeze. I could hardly bear to think about what this young lass had endured those last few weeks – and yet, somehow, she'd found the will to survive.

It was a Saturday, and I rushed her to the out-of-hours vet, expecting the worst. Beside me, Adelaida sat in the passenger seat, filming our journey. I suspected listeriosis, a bacterial infection of the brain, caused by listeria bacteria in spoiled silage, which tracks up cuts in the gums, into the brain, causing encephalitis and abscesses. Essentially, her brain was being eaten away by bacteria, and this had been happening for weeks.

'I'm really not hopeful, Lexy, but we can try antibiotics – really high doses, for three days – and some pain relief. But I don't think she's going to make it . . .'

The vet tried to give me a little ray of hope, but my instinct knew: she was going to die, and the only thing I could do was make her death gentle and peaceful. In the short time she had – maybe a few days, if that – I'd try to replace the loneliness, pain and hopelessness she'd endured, with love, peace and hope. I'll never forget that deep despair eating away at my insides, as I looked at the sheep who wanted to live, knowing that she was going to die. It was painful, right down into my core.

While Isa set up shots, and Adelaida and Scott got into position, I prepared a small part of a shed for her. I heaped it with straw to keep her warm, and put bales around the area to help her hold herself up. I cut up some carrots and broccoli and got her some water, and prepared her antibiotic injection.

'Hey, Maya – look, darling girl! It's all cosy and warm for ye . . . Come on in, sweetheart, let's get ye settled.'

Isa had named her Maya: 'A beautiful name for a beautiful lassie, eh, sweetie?'

Maya could barely walk, but with a little help, she could stand up, and she sometimes managed a few wobbling strides before crashing to the ground. It was hellish to watch, but I had to keep her moving. If she did have any chance of surviving, she'd have to keep using her muscles. As Gimli watched with curiosity from the other side of the fence, trying to work out what was going on, Maya tried so hard to get up and stay up, and every time she fell, she *Maaaa*ed in frustration. I had to be her cheerleader, staying positive and encouraging her to keep going, but my heart was breaking and, in a way, I felt like I was betraying her with lies.

For a couple of days, while Isa, Adelaida and Scott did their thing around us, I sat with Maya in the shed, reading my book and helping her to eat her carrots and broccoli and apple – her favourites. She was a sweet lass, always ready for a cuddle, and she loved having a pal beside her. When she wanted to stand, I'd help her up, and encourage her outside to do her wees and get her exercise. I could see her spirit brought alive by our friendship and I tried hard to keep the tears to myself.

Late on Monday evening, we were filming outside in the glow of the security light. We wanted to capture Maya's determination, and my hopes and fears for her. She was insistent that she was going to walk, and, over the last couple of days, she seemed to have got a little bit stronger.

'Maya . . . Come on, darling, out ye come . . .' I stood outside the shed and egged her on. 'Come on, sweetie, ye can do it!'

With all the might she had, she hauled herself up on wobbly legs and bolted out of the shed. Off she went through the snow, away across the lawn and into the darkness. We all stopped and looked at each other, waiting for the crash and the deflated 'Maaaa'. A few seconds later, she appeared at the other side of the garden. She'd managed a whole lap of the house.

'Oh, Maya, darlin', look at ye! Yer walking!'

She was so pleased with herself. She tottered right past me, determined, heading for her shed. In one go, without stopping, she'd done it. She'd wanted to walk without falling over, and she'd done it.

Sobbing and laughing, I called to my pal from outside the shed. 'Oh, Maya! Ye did it! Ye actually did it!'

'Maaaaaaaaa!' she shouted back, clearly delighted.

She was so pleased with what she'd done. She wanted to live. She was only young, less than a year old, and she had fought so hard for this shot at life. But there was nothing I could do to help her, except be her cheerleader at the end. I could feel the inevitable heartbreak rise inside me, knowing I was powerless to change what had already been set in motion long before we met.

'Right, young lady, that's enough excitement for one day. Let's get you into bed . . .'

The crew had just left and, in the quiet of the late evening, we had a cuddle. She loved her cuddles.

'Ye did it, Maya! Ye did it. A whole lap. Yer amazing, ye know that? Here, I think you've earned this.' I handed her a Hobnob and we sat together for a few minutes while she chewed on her biscuit and I made sure her hay bales were propping her up so she could sit upright. 'Right, darling, it's bedtime. You've had a big day, eh? It's bedtime for us both, I think. I'm so proud of you, sweetheart. I love you. Night night.' I kissed her forehead, turned out the light and left Maya alone.

I didn't know then that would be the last time I'd see her alive. A few hours later, while I was sleeping, the damage to her brain reached its inevitable tipping point, and a devastating seizure ended her life.

Our film, *Crannog*, premiered at the Edinburgh International Film Festival on 21 June 2018. A few of my friends from online and real life were going to see it with us, and I'd arranged for an after-party meal at Seeds for the Soul, a wee local vegan cafe just up the road from the theatre. I thought it was a good excuse for Bran the Man to meet his many online fans, and I'd arranged for him to make a special surprise guest appearance.

After exchanging an arm and a leg for an underground parking space, and getting Bran settled for his couple of hours in the car, I met Mum and Dad outside the car park and, chatting excitedly, we made our way through the crowded city streets, up towards the theatre. I was nervous, and worried that people coming along especially to see it would think I'd messed it up. Outside, a crowd of familiar faces was gathering. It felt surreal that they were there to see a film about me, and how much I loved sheep.

'Beverley! Miriam! Michele! Heather! . . . Jane! Annette! Kate! Hi!' I was absolutely delighted and totally overwhelmed. It was such an honour, and I was starting to understand what imposter syndrome felt like. 'Thanks so much for coming; it's so nice tae see ye! Are ye well?' We hugged and chatted. I was thrilled to bits.

'Right, time to get inside.' Dad, keeping an eye on his watch while I blethered and giggled and lost all sense of responsibility, herded us inside.

Mum and Dad sat behind me, which I found reassuring, and, when I glanced back, Mum looked like she was about to burst. Isa and I sat together, nervously holding hands and clutching our programmes.

Crannog.

Director:	*Isa Rao.*
Run Time:	*15 minutes.*
Synopsis:	*Crannog follows Alexis as she tirelessly tries to nurse a neglected sheep back to health. A quiet reflection on kindness in the face of death, the film intimately explores the fragility and strength that comes from dedicating your life to the care of others.*

It was a huge moment for both of us. We gripped each other as the theatre went dark.

'MaaaaaaaAAA!' shouted Gimli from the screen, and our nerves dissolved into laughter. *The Big Woolly Bastard on the big screen.* I could hardly believe what was happening.

It had been a few months since Maya died, but, together with the excitement and nerves, seeing her again was too much. As soon as the credits rolled, I rushed to the toilets, sobbing. While I was standing over the sink, splashing my face and trying to compose myself, someone from the audience came and stood beside me.

'That was beautiful,' she said. 'That sheep . . . I was so sad when she died. I didn't know sheep had so much personality.'

My face creased into fresh tears. It was really happening. I'd dreamed of this, of being able to show people who sheep really were, how much more there was to them. Maya had fought so hard for the life she was fated never to be able to live, but she was living on, in this theatre, in the hearts and minds of people who had never met her, but who wouldn't forget what she had shown them.

I love you, Maya. We did it, darling. We did it.

On that midsummer night, surrounded by friends in Seeds for the Soul, we ate, blethered, laughed, cried, raised a glass to Maya and her kind, and celebrated. It had been overwhelming and had seemed impossible at times, but we'd done it. Together with Isa and the rest of the team, Maya and I had told her story. We'd shown what love had done for her. We'd shown the world another way.

When Bran made his special appearance, he was greeted with cries of absolute delight. Revelling in the love and good times, he shoogled his way into the cafe, soaking up all the fussing and admiration in the way that only one who knows they totally deserve it can. It was wonderful. This old man, who had been abandoned to wander the streets of that very city, sick and alone, was back there now, wobbly but healthy, master of the universe, and absolutely loving it.

I watched Bran shoogling from fan to fan, grinning like a loon, basking in the love. There was a long way to go and I knew I needed to make some big decisions and changes, but things were happening. I was starting to feel like, somehow, I'd managed to stumble on to the right path.

CHAPTER TWELVE

Somewhere Nice to Live

It was still hard to believe that in just a couple of years, my family and the hospice had outgrown the place I'd gone to fade away and die. The turkey lads had been joined by three turkey ladies, and with each rescue and rehoming day, more hens had joined the flock. Folk had told me about some cockerels who were going to be killed, so a few of them had joined us, too, which unsurprisingly didn't go down too well with my only neighbour. The piglets were meant to be temporary lodgers, but of course they were staying. Then Gimli had joined the party, and you can't just have one sheep – seven was a much better number. It was overcrowded, the land was struggling to cope, and with Bran, B and Ri, our tiny cottage was bursting at the seams, too. Something had to give. Either I stopped in my tracks and found new homes for the piglet lads, cockerels and some of the sheep, or I kept going, expanded, and took the whole thing to the next level.

I was delighted to be alive and to even have the option of moving, but just the thought of trying to find somewhere that was right in all the ways it needed to be – and then moving everyone there – made me want to build a couch fort and hide in it until a grown-up had rectified the situation.

But Bran was too busy shouting into the ether, and Gimli's hooves were no good with a keyboard, so, feeling very much like I did when I was trawling dating sites, I scoured estate-agent sites, day after day, looking for a potential new home. I was still penniless, but Mum and Dad, as supportive as ever of my wild dream chases, offered me my inheritance early. So, combined with what I hoped I'd get for selling the cottage, I had a budget of about £250,000. It was an extraordinary amount to me, beyond anything I'd ever have hoped for, but even with the net cast wide and a willingness to consider anything remotely suitable, there were very few places in my price range. Most houses with the quality of land and acreage that my family needed were way over budget, or the house was a ruin (or non-existent). I needed somewhere that had a house that was at least habitable, with good grazing for the sheep, hard, rocky areas for the pigs and enough space for the chicken and turkey folk. And, perhaps most importantly, I wanted to build a dedicated animal hospice building on the land, too – the first of its kind in the world. Bran had never had a home of his own and I desperately wanted to give him that gift. My dream was to create a warm, cosy space, so that he and B, and any other animals that came along in the future, could live out their last days in comfort. But this long wish list certainly ruled out a semi in the 'burbs.

Day after day, I looked, but there was nothing that ticked the boxes and I was losing the will to live. I was so desperate that I even looked at a house in Campbeltown, a three-hour drive from the mainland, at the end of a peninsula, and at a farm described as 'handy for the West Coast Main Line'. They weren't lying: as Mum and I viewed the living room, the 15:03 to London shot past in a cloud of fumes, about five feet from the window, and just about took Mum's glasses with it.

My enthusiasm had waned about three minutes into the search, but I kept trying. The situation at the cottage was getting more stressful and unmanageable, and something had to give – and soon. I gave myself a time limit of six months; if I'd not found something by then, I'd reassess and very reluctantly consider the other option.

I was about five and a half months in, and on the verge of defeat, when Mum's friends, Linda and Irene – who, unfathomably, love a good house search – found a listing for an old, traditional farmhouse, with four and a half acres, just outside Kirkcudbright, in a hidden corner of south-west Scotland. On paper, Ringliggate looked like it might have what we were looking for, and it was just inside budget. I wasn't holding my breath, though; jaded, despondent and cynical about the whole thing, I was expecting it to go the same way as all the others. To save me the long, point-less journey, Mum and Dad travelled down from Kilmarnock to view it.

'We've found it!' On the other end of the line, Mum was buzzing. 'This is it. This is the one.' Mum and I have always had a feeling for houses; we're both drawn to some, and repelled by others. I wanted to believe her, but I didn't. Still, I wasn't tripping over other options, so I reluctantly arranged to go and see it the following weekend.

On a snowy February day, battling a self-induced tantrum because I got horribly lost and ended up late for the viewing, I stepped into Ringliggate. Mum was right: I felt like I'd come home.

The old house had been neglected, unlived-in and unloved for a long time. It reeked of damp, and the antique boiler and electrics were on the verge of being condemned. Paint was peeling off the crumbling walls and the kitchen had been so badly fitted that the dishwasher was broken and unusable, without ever having cleaned a dish in its life. The land needed as much attention as the house in order to get it into a decent enough state for animals to live on it.

Even if I'd known about the surprises still to come – the pond under the dining-room floor and the mushrooms growing out of the chimney breast – they wouldn't have been enough to put me off. It needed a lot of love to warm up its bones and I'd need to put it back together from the inside out, but finally, I'd found our new home. On 30 April 2018, I collected the keys to Ringliggate, and to our new life.

The move from Ballindalloch, in the Highlands, down to the opposite end of the country was overwhelmingly daunting and had far too much margin for error, for my liking. There was an almost incomprehensible amount of work to do: a hospice to build, a sanctuary to create – and I needed to raise the money to do it all, too. Though it was in one piece and had a functioning toilet and kitchen, the house needed a lot of work to sort out the damp and make it safely habitable. Up at the cottage, there was a lot that needed to be done to make it sellable, even before four piglets and a very naughty chicken had played at *Extreme Makeover: Home Edition* in it. Now, after their 'help', we were looking at a partial rebuild. The only option was for Dad to take out a bridging loan to enable me to buy Ringliggate while getting the cottage into something resembling a sellable state.

Within days of getting the keys to Ringliggate, I hired a local company to get to work on the sanctuary fencing, while up in Ballindalloch, I moved into the caravan and started focusing on raising the funds I needed to pay for it all. I wanted the land to be as safe as it could be for the bird folk, and it was important to me that they had a home where they could make their own decisions. With that in mind, I chose to get the entire four and a half acres circled in a predator-proof fence. It was going to be six feet high, dug down two feet into the ground, and it would have an overhang to stop foxes and mink being able to get in. I figured that, with the fence keeping them safe, if the cockerels wanted to have a bachelor pad in a gorse bush, or if the turkey ladies wanted to sleep out in the long grass in summer, then they could, and I'd be able to sleep sound, too. It was going to cost £25,000, though, and trying to get people excited about donating for a fence wasn't easy. Vital as it was, it wasn't exactly the sexiest of fundraising campaigns.

Meanwhile, the foundations for the hospice needed to be dug, filled and levelled before the sections of the building I'd commissioned arrived. With extraordinary kindness, Dick – the local farmer, whose family had worked the land in the area for generations – offered to do the job, and within hours, he'd sent round some of his workers with an excavator.

I'd been worried about how my slightly unusual family was going to be accepted by the local community. I'd never felt very settled in Ballindalloch; as much as I loved the cottage, I always felt like a bit of an outsider. I tentatively hoped we'd fit in with our new neighbours and eventually be part of the community, but very quickly I felt warmly welcomed. I was overwhelmed by the kindness and help that Dick and Stuart, his shepherd, offered, and within hours of getting the keys, Mandy and Sam next door had popped round to let me know to just shout if I needed anything.

As work to bring order to Ringliggate progressed, up in the cottage, things were utter chaos. What had been left in the post-piglet kitchen wasteland was ripped out, and the living room was stripped back to bare walls and floors. A toaster, kettle and wee halogen oven, set up on an old bit of worktop in the living room, did their best to provide adequate meals. There was no hot water and no washing machine, and I did the dishes in the bath.

Life in the caravan was hot, smelly and cramped, but it had its upsides. I loved being almost outside with the animals, and I felt closer to them in a lot of ways. Gimli and co quickly realised that an open caravan window meant the possibility that it might be a magic Rich-Tea-dispensing window, just like the magic Rich-Tea-dispensing letter box. Every so often, while I was sitting tearing my hair out over the latest *awfurfuckssake* moment involving the move, a pair of sheep lugs would appear at the window, quickly followed by a very distinguished Roman nose and wide, Rich-Tea-addicted eyes.

'Oh, hi Gim.'

'MaaaaaAAAAAAA.'

'Sorry, dude, I don't have any biscuits.'

'MaaaaaAAAAAAAAAAA.'

'But there's nae biscuits, Gim . . .'

'MaaaaaAAAAAAAAAAAAAAAAA.'

'Right, fine: there's biscuits . . .'

As well as the planning, organising, building work, fundraising and everything else that had to be done for the move, the daily care of everyone in the sanctuary and hospice carried on. One afternoon, I'd gone to Elgin to buy stuff for the renovation and some food for everyone. Rushing, I'd got home just in time to collect Elisa, a partially sighted sheep lass, Bran and a hen named Ri Junior, for a three-in-one trip to the vet. I didn't have time to fully unpack the car, so I shoved everyone in as best I could around bags of food, pipe fittings and a stainless-steel sink I'd bought for the new kitchen, and legged it to Grantown.

Check-ups complete, I was loading Elisa back into the boot of the car outside the vet clinic, when, confused and a bit alarmed, she let out a loud, protesting, 'Maaaaaaaaaaa.' A couple walking past did a double take, as I held Elisa back and brought the boot down, then they stopped and turned back.

'Is that a . . . sheep?' asked the guy, possibly wondering if this was a new breed of woolly, baaing dog he'd only just discovered. A sheep-dog, if you will.

'Aye, this is Elisa.' I smiled, opening the boot again.

He peered in and Elisa started investigating his face with her nostrils. Bran was in the back seat, wondering why someone else was getting attention and not him.

'And is that a dog in there, too?'

'Aye, that's Bran. He's about 146 years old.'

'Bukkk-uuuuk,' added Ri Junior.

'Was that a . . . chicken?'

By this point, I wasn't sure if I was making this guy's day or making him question his sanity.

'Well, I've never seen the like. You've got everything but the kitchen sink in there . . .'

I opened the back door and moved Bran's blanket to reveal the sink I'd bought a few hours beforehand.

'You've got to be kidding me . . .'

That summer is a bit of a blur, partly because of some self-preservation mechanism that has kicked in to stop me ever having to experience that shit show again, and partly because of the horrible brain fog that I just wasn't able to shake off. There were some really good, memorable times: shearing the sheep in Dad's trailer with my friends Gill and Jim, over a couple of sweaty, hilarious days, in thirty-degree heat; and finding my old wedding dress while packing, and doing the rounds wearing it with my wellies, one evening, with Gimli as my bridesmaid. But mostly it was frustrating, worrying, daunting, overwhelming, soul-destroying, and whatever was going wrong with my body was making me wonder if I was dying.

'Aye,' was the answer. 'Pretty much.'

One hot, sweaty, delirious afternoon in July, I collapsed on to the grubby, worn-out caravan bed. My muscles had seized up and my bones ached with pains that shot up and through them like needles of fire. I felt like someone had opened my veins and drained me of every drop of blood and energy, and like a barely animated stone statue, I lay there, unable to move. My guts gurgled and groaned, and spasms of crippling pain radiated out through me from just above my right hip. I've no idea how long I lay there, barely conscious, thinking that this was how and where I was going to die, and I've no idea how I did the evening rounds that night.

I didn't have time for my body to decide that this was the moment it was going to pack it in. I still had tens of thousands of pounds to raise to pay for the new infrastructure, a move to organise and dozens of animals to look after, but nothing was working anymore. My brain was so foggy I could barely form a sentence, my joints and bones were rippling with agonising shards of angry pain, I could barely stand up, let alone walk, and my guts felt like they were disintegrating inside me.

I don't remember getting to hospital or the first few days of being there. Tests showed another blockage, a bad one, worse than I'd had before. The other symptoms were – and still are – a mystery, but from experience, I now think it was probably exhaustion and stress. While Dad looked after everyone at home, I stayed in hospital, where they filled me with steroids until the inflammation receded a bit, and booked me in for more tests down in Dumfries Royal, in a few weeks, once I'd moved.

By the time I was sent home, I was far from well, but I was feeling a bit less like I was about to keel over. I really hadn't liked being away from everyone, and I was delighted to be heading home to be with my family again. All week, I'd imagined a slow-mo reunion scene with Gimli, the two of us falling into each other's arms in joy.

As soon as I arrived, I ran towards him, ecstatic, and threw my arms around his neck. 'Gimli!' I scattered kisses all over his face and nose, and on the soft bit between his eye and his ear. 'I missed you, pal.' I smiled with relief, feeling better than I had for weeks.

But I wasn't getting the welcome I'd expected. He was cold and aloof, not his usual loving, head-nuzzling self.

'What's the matter, Gim? Dad, has he been OK?'

He'd been fine, Dad told me, but a bit quieter than normal.

Crouching beside him, I felt a pull on my leg that almost toppled me over. Gim had hoisted one of his front legs and hooked it over my thigh. He was pulling me in, closer to him, as close as he could get me.

'Gim, what you doing, son?' I laughed, trying to keep my balance. But I knew exactly what he was telling me.

Where do ye think you've been? I cannae trust you, wummin. You're staying here, even if I have to make sure of it myself . . .

*

I had six weeks left to organise the move and fund the ongoing hospice build. In a blur of letters begging for raffle prizes, fund-raisers organised by supporters, online campaigns via Facebook, pleas in the local paper, sweat and tears and meltdowns, by the end of July, I'd scraped together more than £80,000. It was incredible and I was overwhelmed – with gratitude, utter relief and exhaustion. The fencing was done, the chicken sheds were in place and the pig paddocks were ready. The hospice building itself was there, but it was still an empty shell. In my head, I knew exactly what I wanted it to look like. I imagined it was going to be a warm, welcoming home, somewhere that B and Bran and the folk who came to live there in the future would be comfortable and safe. I didn't want it to be cold, clinical or medical. I wanted them to have cosy bedrooms, outdoor patios, a living room, a kitchen and a wet room, and plenty of space to potter outside. But I was running out of time, and even with what seemed like the huge amount I'd raised, there was so much to be done, money was already getting tight. I focused on getting bedrooms ready for Bran and B, and the rest would have to come later.

Move day finally arrived. Hard as the summer had been, this was the bit I was dreading the most. The stress of moving everyone 300 miles to the other end of the country hung over me, but thankfully, a friend I'd met online, Alan, had recently bought an ex-livestock truck specifically so that he could fill the transport gap for sanctuaries, who always struggle to find suitable ways to move larger animals. For us, the timing couldn't have been better, and I think we were either his first or his second 'customer'.

With paperwork, movement certificates and everything else in place, Alan and the truck pulled into the drive. We'd decided to move the pigs on the first day, and everyone else – sheep, chickens, turkeys and dogs – on the second. The hot, dry weather we'd had all summer had broken a few days before, and the cool breeze was a welcome relief and a weight off my mind, because I'd been worried about how everyone would cope in the heat on the long journey. Unfortunately, the torrential downpours that had freshened everything up and cleared the muggy air had also softened the top layer of earth, and within seconds of pulling on to the grass, the truck was stuck fast.

It took an hour under the truck, a lot of swearing and a frantic dash to find someone local with a tractor to get us out, but a couple of hours later than planned, a remarkably calm Alan set off. Emily, Charlotte, Barnaby, Brian, Carl and Andrew were on their way to their new home.

The next day, things started off a bit more smoothly. Apart from a couple of renegade escapees, who'd made the executive decision that there was no bloody way they were going in those crates, the rest of the chickens and the turkeys were loaded into crates and secured in the truck. Sheep are a lot more cooperative and a lot less likely to turn someone into a human pancake than pigs, so getting them on the truck was sure to be a lot less stressful than loading the pigs had been, the day before. But, of course, there had to be someone who threw a spanner in the works. As we were luring the sheep up the ramp, I noticed that Hazel wasn't barging everyone out of the way to get to the bucket of food. If

Hazel wasn't at the front of the food queue, there was definitely, without a doubt, something wrong.

'Hang on . . . Where's Hazel?' Panic rising, I started to search.

Eventually, I found her, lying in a corner of the garden, looking forlorn.

I rushed over to her. 'What's the matter, darling?'

Her head was hanging low, and not even a biscuit was tempting her.

I could feel my adrenaline starting to flow – something was really wrong.

Leaving Alan to it in a flurry of apologies, I hoisted Hazel's enormous woolly arse into the car and rushed to the vet.

Waiting anxiously outside the farmed animal examination room, I chewed my nails and tried to say calm, but I was really worried. I couldn't bear the thought of something happening to Hazel; she was barcly a year old, and she was one hundred per cent sass. The door opened and the vet appeared, taking off his gloves.

'Is Hazel . . . quite, um . . . spoiled? Maybe not used to being . . . a wee bit sore?' I could see a smile on his lips.

Frowning, confused, I thought about it. 'Well, aye, I guess she is a bit spoiled . . . She's got it pretty good, I suppose, and she is a bit of a drama queen.'

'Aye. I thought so. She's just grazed her knee; she'll be fine.'

As Alan secured the back door of the truck and got on his way, I loaded the car up with my last few things and, with drama queen Hazel and Bran, we set off on our journey south. Dad was staying behind with Ri and B for a few more days, to do the last of the work on the cottage – and catch some AWOL chickens – but I was leaving for the last time. In the drama of the morning, I'd barely had time to take it in. I'd not had time to go and visit the graveyard in the woods where Georgia and all her friends were buried, and I'd not had a chance to go and sit on Maggie's mound, the place where she used to sit and watch over her garden that she loved so much. The cottage had brought Maggie so much joy, and now I was leaving behind the last place that we'd shared and made memories together. I imagined how much Mags would have loved exploring all the nooks and crannies of Ringliggate. My heart lurched. Ahead of me, the truck started to pull away. I took a deep breath and gathered my strength. It hurt like hell, but life couldn't stand still. Maggie would always be with me and I was going to make sure that her legacy lived on.

It was after dark and the summer rain was lashing sideways when we finally arrived, stressed and exhausted. I still felt awful, and the long drive on top of the worry, pressure and toil of the last few days had wiped me out. As the rain came down in sheets, Mum, Alan and I slipped and stumbled through the mud by torchlight, unloading everyone from the truck. While I coaxed the sheep through the new gates and into their field, Mum and Alan unloaded the crates of stressed, worried chickens into their sheds. Battling against the mud, cramps seized me and I screamed in pain as muscles I didn't know I had tightened and clenched in hot, burning flashes. I was starving, but eating was excruciating, and I knew anything I ate would come straight back up again, anyway. I'd had a fair few emergency stops in lay-bys on the way down, as my guts gurgled and spasmed.

With everyone settled, Alan set off on his journey home, probably glad to see the back of us. He'd done a brilliant job, and he deserved a well-earned rest. Mum and I shook ourselves off in the kitchen and put the kettle on. I was ready for a long sleep and a bit of a rest tomorrow.

Tomorrow . . .

'Aw, shit, I've just remembered!' Wide-eyed, I stared at Mum in horror. 'I've got a live radio interview in Dumfries at eleven o'clock tomorrow morning.'

The interview went really well, and a few days later, a journalist called Joan got in touch to ask if I'd like to share the story of the hospice with her. She'd caught part of the interview on the radio and she was intrigued by the idea, and she wanted to pitch it to some national newspapers. The following week, Gimli and I were posing, up on the hillside, doing a photo shoot for the *Guardian*.

Everyone was settling in, and the chickens, turkeys, pigs and sheep loved their new homes. Bran was finding it a bit difficult to settle into his new bedroom, and of course, there was only one solution to that: incessant barking. Very quickly, visitors started arriving, keen to see our new pad. A few volunteers came to stay in those first few weeks, too, which was a great help while I struggled to set everything up and cope with the enormity of the daily tasks.

In late September, the *Guardian* article came out. Sitting at the dining-room table with Sara, a volunteer who'd been staying for a couple of weeks, we couldn't keep up with the phone calls and emails, which started at seven a.m. and continued all day. Media enquiries came from the BBC, ITV, local newspapers, national newspapers, China, Greece and Ohio. I had no idea what was happening and I was completely overwhelmed.

But while all this exciting stuff was going on, my body was failing again. I could barely eat, sleep or control my bowels, and cramps and spasms grasped and gnawed at my muscles and intestines. One night, I fell asleep leaning on the open door of the grill, waiting for food I wouldn't eat to cook. I knew something was going badly wrong, and I knew I had to slow down, but I didn't have time. I had to keep going.

On an overcast day in mid-October, my body took the dilemma out of my hands. Trudging through mud on my way to do the morning rounds, a bolt of pain like nothing I'd ever felt shot through me, and I doubled over, groaning into the mud. *Oh no . . .*

CHAPTER THIRTEEN

Alive and Breathing

'Right, let's see if we can get it in, this time.' The nurse consoled me as she adjusted the needle, trying to find a vein.

'Fuuuuuuucccckkkk . . . Please . . . please, make it stop . . .' I groaned and gripped her hand as another shock of pain rippled through me.

'It's OK, darling, we're getting there. Don't worry, we're going to get some morphine in you soon.' My veins were never the most cooperative, and sometimes getting anything into or out of them was almost impossible.

I'd been well acquainted with pain over the last fifteen years, but I'd never known anything like this. Every few seconds, a spasm gripped and twisted my intestines, sending shards of pain through the inflamed, raw tissue. It started just above my right hip, in a dull pulsating throb, which built and got more intense, until it radiated out through my intestines, every spasm more painful than the last. With each grabbing and twisting, I winced and clenched, doubling over, moaning, pleading for it to stop. Within a minute or so, it had reached its crescendo, then it would suddenly stop, as if someone had flicked a switch, and I'd release and unclench, breathless, frozen in terror as I braced myself and waited for the next dull throb, and the whole thing would start again.

You know the scene in *Alien*, where John Hurt falls back on to the dining table and the chestbuster erupts out of his guts? The screenwriter, Dan O'Bannon, had Crohn's, and he wrote that scene into the movie because he said that the pain of Crohn's felt like an alien in your guts, ripping at your insides, trying to eat its way out. Aye. What he said.

'Right, darling, that's us in. Here we go, let's get this in you.'

The cool liquid started snaking its way up my vein.

'Aw, thank fuck . . . Thank you . . .' As the morphine hit, I sank back on the pillow into painless bliss. I could have hugged the nurse, Nikki – that wonderful lady with the magic needle that takes the pain away. I probably did. We're still friends on Facebook.

Unsurprisingly, I don't remember anything about the next few hours. It was dark when I woke up in my bed in the ward, and it took me a few seconds to work out where I was and put the pieces together. The morphine was wearing off, and I could feel the pain as an echo, low in my right-hand side. I lightly pressed the flesh above the bit where the pain was coming from. Bloody hell, that hurt. I didn't know exactly what was going on, but I strongly suspected it was a blockage or rupture of some sort. Whatever it was, it was bad.

I eased myself out of bed and slowly walked to the toilet. Wincing, I unpacked my toothbrush and toothpaste from my backpack, brushed my teeth and then crawled back into bed. It was just after three a.m. Sleep wasn't going to come easy. I opened my laptop.

Awfurfuckssake . . .

Apparently, in my opiate-induced delirium, I'd decided that I was an artist, now, and that my new-found 'talent' should be shared with the world. There, on the hospice page, was my portrait of Charles, the dickhead turkey, which looked a bit like a pissed-off dodo wearing an assortment of male-genital-related paraphernalia from a hen party on its head. Seemingly, Gimli was a nurse from the 1940s, now, too – *Sister B. W. B'Stard*, his name badge told me – and he had a wee white hat with a red cross, and a stethoscope. I'd posted his portrait, too, and told everyone that he was going to look after me while I was in hospital. As well as seeing that I'd got off my nut and embarrassed myself on social media, I also found a lot of really nice messages and well wishes from friends and hospice supporters, sending love and hoping that I'd be on the mend and back home soon.

Home.

How was everyone? Had they all had their dinner and gone to bed on time? Dad was at the hospice, taking care of things, but I didn't like not being there. Before I'd left, I'd limped round to see everyone, just in case. B, Hazel, Hilary, the turkey ladies, Elisa, the piglet lads, Gimli, Bran, Ri . . .

I closed my laptop, took off my glasses and tried to get comfortable. In the dead of night, with things beeping and clicking and puffing around me, I wondered if this might be the time the Crohn's finally defeated me.

Nope.

I had to see my family again. I had to believe I was going to get better and go home. Anything else wasn't an option.

As soon as they could, Mum and Dad came to see me. I was being filled with drugs to control the pain and tackle the inflammation, and I don't remember much about them being there, but I hazily remember them sitting by my bed, Dad looking worried, Mum crying and holding my hand and whispering something in my ear about a trip to Brighton to eat ourselves silly for a week, once I was better.

Fortuitously, a few days before I collapsed, I'd had the MRI that had been arranged when I was in hospital in Elgin. Because I couldn't eat much, I'd become underweight and anaemic, so I'd also had an iron transfusion the week before. The consultant had suspected a planned surgery might be on the horizon, and they wanted to make sure I was ready for it. Without knowing it, I'd been prepared for the surgery it was now looking likely I was going to need.

When the gastrointestinal surgeon and the surgical registrar came to see me, to go over what they'd discovered from the recent MRI, the upshot was that it was looking pretty grim in there. The bit of my intestine that had been so badly damaged before –

the holey mass of diseased tissue that had threatened to bump me off, three years before – had finally reached its end game. It was a sticky, gnarly, inflamed, blocked, rupturing mess. Worse, it had started to stick itself to my kidney and urethra, and to my abdominal wall. It needed to come out – soon.

'There's no doubt that you need surgery,' the consultant said. 'But there are some problems. With your kidney and abdomen involved, it's made it a lot more complicated and risky.'

He was a compassionate, serious, respectful young guy, and I instinctively trusted him. He explained that he was going to speak to his colleagues in urology, and to the inflammatory bowel disease team. There would need to be a urology surgeon there during the operation, too, and they'd need to stent my kidney and urethra to protect them as they disentangled them from the sticky mess.

'Being honest, there's a chance that we won't be able to do the surgery,' he told me. 'But we'll do what we can.'

I didn't need to ask what would happen if they couldn't.

As I waited to hear what the doctors had decided they could do for me – or not – the inflammation died down and the morphine wore off, and I started to feel less woozy. The nurses were exceptionally kind, and every hour or so, someone came by to ask me if I needed anything, if I was comfortable, if there was anything they could do for me. Every room in the new Dumfries Royal was private, and although I hated being away from my family, after the relentlessness of the last few months, it was actually quite nice to have nothing to do but lie in bed, in my own little room, with my puzzles, music and books, chatting to folk online – and not

209

pursuing a career as an artist. I wanted for nothing, except my family, back home.

That night, a nurse came to measure me up for a colostomy bag, in case they needed to fit one during surgery. As I stood, holding up my gown, she drew circles on me with a Sharpie and told me that about eighty-five per cent of patients needed the bags when they had this stage of the disease, and this kind of surgery. She promised me that I'd barely notice it; it was really easy to use and it wasn't at all uncommon, and she told me not to worry if I woke up from surgery and found I had one.

At around midday on Thursday, two days after I'd staggered into A & E, the surgeon came back to see me. They'd had the meeting to discuss my situation and what could be done about it.

'Based on what we've found, and what urology have said, I believe I can do the surgery. It's going to be long and compli-cated, but I think I have the experience to do it, if you'll let me.' He looked a bit apprehensive; I liked this guy. 'But I have to warn you,' he said, 'it's going to be a dangerous procedure, and there's a reasonable chance you won't survive.'

'Huh.' I didn't really have much to add to that bombshell.

'Now, I can do it today, or I can do it on Monday, when I'm back on shift. If you want to do it today, I'll cancel the elective surgeries this afternoon and we'll get you down to the theatre. If you want some time to think about it, we can wait until Monday.' He paused. 'But you don't have much longer than that.'

'Huh.'

'Take your time. I know it's a lot to take in.' He sat down on the window ledge to give me a moment to think. Behind him, the Galloway Hills stretched into the distance.

'So, if I don't have the surgery, I'll be dead by next week?'

He paused, and nodded.

'I guess we better get a move on, then.'

He smiled. 'Great. I'll see you downstairs in an hour.'

I looked down at my laptop bag and the corner of my diary sticking out of it. I had so much to do. Things had been so busy with the media interviews and settling into our new home, I'd fallen behind with admin stuff – like donation thank-you emails, replying to messages, Pounds for Poundies, Christmas merchandise and a thousand other things. There was more media coverage coming up soon; a couple of small film crews had been to record short pieces about the hospice and sanctuary, and I wanted to get the new website finished before they aired. I'd been doing some work on it that morning, and there was something that had been bugging me that I hadn't been able to fix. I reached for my laptop. It would only take me a few minutes; I could get it done before I went down to theatre . . . I laughed. *So, this is what you think about when you might only have an hour to live? Fuck's sake.* I put my laptop back in its bag, and called Mum.

I hated how much worry my disease caused my parents. I hadn't always told them every detail, but we'd always faced it together and I knew they would support me through anything. Now, more than ever, they didn't need the gritty details; it wouldn't have helped anything, and they were worried enough.

'We'll see you tomorrow,' sniffed Mum. 'And remember, when this is all over, we're going to Brighton.'

'Bloody right we are! OK, I better go and get ready. They'll call you when I'm out of theatre. Don't worry. I'll see you tomorrow. Mwah-wah.'

'Mwah . . . wa . . .' she almost managed in reply.

I took a deep breath and sat down on the edge of my bed. I looked out of the window, across the car park and over to the hills, and thought about everyone back at home. I checked the time: it was almost half twelve. I'd have finished my rounds by now, and everyone would be fed, clean and enjoying their day.

I called Dad and gave him the gist of it. He'd been expecting the news, and he was worried, but pragmatic. I could hear the cockerels shouting in the background. Bran had been out for a potter in the garden, and Dad and B had been out for their walk, up to the weather station at the top of the hill. Everyone was happy and well.

'How's Gimli?' I smiled. *Sister B. W. B'stard.*

'He's fine. He's in a huff, though. I think you're in the bad books again.'

I knew I'd be going down to theatre soon, but I felt completely calm. If I was going to die, there seemed no point fighting it. I wanted to see everyone again, but if it was time, it was time. I'd seen so many of my animal pals go through the same thing. I'd looked into their eyes as they'd left this world, and they were so calm and accepting of it. I'd learned from watching them that there was no use fighting it; there was nothing I could do about

212

it. Having faced death a lot, I wasn't scared of it, because I'd seen how peaceful it could be.

Just after one o'clock, a porter arrived. He wheeled me down, helped me up on to a bed in a curtained bay and wished me good luck. There was a lot going on around me, and I felt like the calm eye in the storm. So many people were preparing for this surgery, quickly dashing from the nurses' station to the theatre, and to other places I couldn't see. There were people in light green scrubs, dark green scrubs, blue scrubs, with disposable aprons and gloves, carrying things, moving things. I know they were doing their jobs, but it was a marvel to think that they were doing all this for me, and for every other person who needed surgery to make them better. I was incredibly lucky even to have this chance, and I was determined to get through this, to get better and get home.

The curtain opened and a nurse came in to ask me some questions. Name. Address. Date of birth . . .

'Great, let's get you through to see the anaesthetists.' She beamed, reassuring me, and wheeled me to another cubicle.

After a rundown of the options, the two jolly anaesthetists and I decided on an epidural for the post-surgery pain relief. It made me squirm just thinking about it, but I figured, if I thought I'd been in pain before, I'd not experienced being sliced open down the middle, having bits of me cut out, and then being stapled back together again. I'd no desire to be in pain ever again, so, icky as it was, I told them to get that thing in my spine. They pulled the curtain round the cubicle and left to fetch what they needed.

213

Having the epidural put in is something I never want to think about or relive again. Still reeling, I was wheeled through to theatre, where a warm, kind nurse helped me up on to the operating table. Everything was brand new and shiny, and I felt like I was on the set of *Star Trek*. I could see the anaesthetists nearby, ready with their syringes, but I couldn't see the surgeon among the rest of the folk rushing past and around each other.

'Right, darlin', that's us. We're ready.' The nurse leaned over me, beaming kindness down on me, and gently lifted my glasses off my face.

Without warning, a wave of panic rushed up. *Shit shit shit.*

'Am I going to be OK?' I pleaded.

She took my hand in hers and I gripped her, fear seizing me.

'You're going to be just fine, darlin'. She smiled, and squeezed my hand. 'We're going to start counting backwards from ten, OK? Ready? Ten . . . nine . . .'

Elisa . . . Hazel . . . Charles . . . Georgia . . . eight . . . Mum . . . Dad . . . Angus . . . Ri . . . Annie . . . seven . . . B . . . Gimli . . . six . . . Maggie . . . five . . . Bran . . .

'Grrrrrgggh hgggh grmmmgh . . .'

'Hi, darlin'. It's OK. You've had an operation. Try to lie still.'

I tried to lift my hand to my face. Something was . . . there . . .

'Try to rest.' The nurse gently took my hand and held it in hers, and I felt the warmth of her skin on my cold fingers. 'You just sleep, darlin'. I'll make sure you're OK.'

The next few days were brutal. There were wires and needles, and I had a tube down my throat to help empty the acid from my stomach and stop me feeling nauseous, and it made me gag every time I swallowed. My guts were still paralysed in shock at what had just happened to them, and the only sustenance I could have was a few sips of water every now and then. The epidural was controlling the pain, and the only thing I could do was lie there and drift in and out of sleep, and hold on to the thought that this would pass, I'd come through it and I'd be home soon.

I'd prepared myself for the prospect of waking up with a colostomy bag; it was more likely than not, and it wasn't something that really bothered me. I'd actually rather empty a bag a few times a day than run to the toilet thirty times, with all the discomfort and embarrassment and loss of dignity that went along with it. But, as it turned out, I was bagless.

When they'd opened me up, they'd taken out the rotten bit and, with the help of a marble (yes, a marble), they'd found a few other small scar-tissue blockages along the length of my intestine. They sliced them open, stitched them inside out and sewed them back up again. Apart from that, my intestines were actually in pretty good shape. There was no sign of active disease, and what had, for years, been angry, raw, diseased tissue was now healthy and pink, and I'd avoided a bag.

I was determined to get through it, though, and my mind, as always, was on the hospice and all I had to do. The day after my surgery, sitting in bed at two a.m. in critical care, crying with frustration, I finally worked out the problem I'd been having with the website. I managed to fix it – just in time for the release

215

of the article about the hospital that was being published that morning.

Mum and Dad visited when they could, and I got regular updates from home. Everyone was fine, but Gimli's huff was intensifying by the day. Bran was wondering where I was, too; Dad was taking care of him, but it wasn't the same as having his wummin. I was going to have a lot of making up to do, when I got home.

Sometime that week, my friend Karen and her mum Berda made their way from Kilmarnock to come to visit me. Berda was really ill herself, and she'd recently started using a wheelchair. I don't even remember the details now, but in typical Karen and Berda fashion, something ridiculous, embarrassing and hilarious had happened on their way there, and we spent the afternoon in hysterics. Karen was, once again, exactly what I needed, and I laughed until I ached.

A couple of weeks before I'd gone into hospital, I'd had a call to tell me that I'd been nominated for the Great Scot Community Champion Award, run by the *Daily Record*. You were nominated and voted for by the public, and I was thrilled. After finding out about my nomination, I shared the post and asked if anyone would like to vote for me and the hospice. It would be great for the hospice, and – I can't deny – an ego boost for me if I won, but I was up against two other folk who were doing great work for their communities in Scotland, so it really was anyone's game.

The winner would be announced at an award ceremony at a hotel in Glasgow – nine days after my surgery. I knew there was no way I was going to make it, and I was a bit gutted (pardon the pun) at the timing, but it was what it was.

A few days before the announcement, however, I got a call from the lady organising the awards do. She was lovely, and she was doing her best to arrange for me to be there by video link, so I could watch the ceremony from my hospital bed. She said she had some news.

'I'm not supposed to do this, and you have to promise not to tell anyone . . . but we've counted the votes, and you've won. You're our Community Champion for 2018.'

'No way.' I laughed. 'For real?'

'Aye, and I had to let you know, in case there is any way you can be there. I know you probably won't be able to, but just in case . . .'

'I'll be there!' I laughed. 'Bloody right, I will be!'

It took some persuasion, and I wasn't beneath using a bit of begging and some *Oh, please – I've won an award* leverage, but I managed to convince the surgeon to wangle me an early release. I'd been doing physio every day and pushing myself as much as I could, without being daft about it, trying to build my strength, and I was pretty steady on my feet. The tubes and wires were all gone, and though I was still stapled up the middle, dosed up to the eyeballs on opiates, and, as my intestines started to slowly and grudgingly wake up again, I felt like I was being skewered by a hot poker every time I tried to eat or go to the toilet, all things considered, I was doing pretty well. I was ready to go home.

It was hard to know how to show my gratitude to the folk who had saved my life and cared for me and been my cheerleaders

NO LIFE TOO SMALL

as I gagged and vomited and wept and raged, and who came rushing when I needed help to restore my balance and dignity in the bathroom at three a.m. I couldn't have asked for more, and I'll be forever grateful.

Eight days after surgery, clutching on to Dad, I wobbled out of the front doors of Dumfries Royal and into the fresh air. I took a deep breath, turned to Dad and smiled. I was alive, and I had a party to go to.

'Look at you!' I laughed as Dad came down the stairs adjusting his bow tie. I'd never seen him in a tux before. He was my plus one for the evening, and my chauffeur, medicine dispenser and holder-upper.

We were almost ready to go. Mum had dug out my grad ball dress, a maroon bias-cut gown, with a cowl neck and a low, plunging back. I hadn't worn it since I was twenty, but it slipped on perfectly, which was just as well, as it was the only posh dress I had. Mum and Dad's neighbour, Claire, who had her own hairdressing business, had come over to do my hair, while Mum painted my toenails to match my dress, and I nibbled at some toast and groaned as my intestines protested. I was so relieved to be out of hospital and back to the familiar.

Hair done, nails painted and make-up on, I slipped into four-inch stilettos, wrapped a fleece around my shoulders, and Dad and I set off.

They'd arranged that I could arrive late in the ceremony and sneak into an empty chair near the door, just before the winner of the Great Scot Award was announced. The lady organising the ceremony came to meet us in the foyer.

'You must be so proud of Alexis,' she beamed, as she led us slowly across the slippery marble floor. 'She really deserves to have won this award, especially after all she's been through.'

Dad stopped in his tracks.

'You already know you've won?' He was caught between delight and affront.

'Aye,' I laughed. 'But I promised I wouldnae tell anyone ...' Smiling, I put my arm through his and we made our way to our seats.

I remember standing on the stage and the bright lights, and apparently I gave a speech, but I've no idea what I said. The audience had been told that I'd just had major surgery, so I can only hope they were as forgiving of my attempts at a speech as the hospice supporters were of my attempts at art.

Backstage, clutching my award, I did the photo shoot, hand-shakes and small talk, and I remember everyone being really kind to me. As we were doing the last of the photos, my guts gurgled as they finally started to rouse from their slumber. Grimacing, I smiled through the pain. I was delighted to have won, and thrilled to be alive and breathing and out of hospital and wearing a fancy frock, but in that moment, I'd have handed that award back in a second in exchange for a good fart.

Back in the car, I got my heels off and my hoodie on. Dad wrapped the fleece round my shoulders, smiling.

'You knew you'd won?' He shook his head. 'Ready for home?'

I was exhausted, and ready for bed, in my old bedroom, with my old wallpaper and all the familiar smells and sounds of home.

A rumble came up from my guts. It had been weeks since I'd last eaten proper solid food. I was ready. It was time. There was only one thing for it.

'Aye,' I said. 'But can we go and get some chips first?'

CHAPTER FOURTEEN

B-Bop-a-Loo-Bop-a-Woppa-Bamma-Boom

I staggered forwards towards the sink, grasped the rim and crumpled.

'*Bloody hell . . .*'

I'd been home at Ringliggate for a couple of days. I wasn't supposed to climb the stairs, so I was under strict instructions to stay upstairs while my family and friends rallied round to look after everyone, including me. I felt pretty much like I'd expect to feel after almost dying, being knocked out, cut open, taken apart a bit and stapled back together, but I was very glad to be home.

I was too weak and too likely to injure myself or get an infection to go outside and see everyone, but I could look out of the bathroom window to the hospice and sanctuary. For a few minutes a day, I propped myself up on the windowsill and watched everyone pottering around in the ebbing light of the last days of autumn: the sheep folk quietly munching on the hillside; the drama of the daily chicken soap opera; the pigs, up on the rocky outcrop at the back of the sanctuary, rooting around, doing their excavations. I didn't need to look out the bathroom window to know where Bran was; I could hear him from my bedroom, with the windows closed.

I looked over to the half-finished hospice building and thought about how much work there was still to do. It was wonderful seeing it there, a real, tangible thing, something that, a few months ago, had just been a thought and a dream. There were problems with the building, though, and a very long snagging list. There was no running water, and I had to run an extension cable from the house to get power. It still wasn't the home I'd imagined for Bran and B, but I couldn't expect everything to happen at once, and they both had warm, safe bedrooms and plenty of space outside to potter. It would get better, it would come together eventually, and I was looking forward to seeing them both enjoying it when it was a proper, finished home for them.

An ache shivered through me; time to go back to bed. I hated lying in bed, incapable, bored and restless. When I'd had so much to do I could cry, all I'd wanted was to go to bed and sleep. Now that I'd been instructed to go to bed and sleep, all I wanted was to have so much to do I could cry.

I was still taking painkillers, but it was over-the-counter stuff rather than the opiates I'd been given in hospital, and there wasn't a bit of me that wasn't aching. The staples were there for another week or so, and as my scar started to heal round them, it was getting itchy and sore. Twinges still spasmed through me as my intestines adjusted to the new floorplan, and pain shot through the bits of intestine that had been bruised and battered and stitched back together. I wanted to be better *now*, and I was trying to push myself towards it a bit more every day. I forced myself to eat, knowing that, two hours later, it'd pass over the scar tissue like crushed glass.

I felt weak for a long time as my muscles starved and went unused, and I felt like I was dragging rather than carrying my body around. I wanted to take the chance to build it back up stronger, so I tried to do an extra physio exercise each day, or just get up and about and keep moving. In the bath, I did Pilates, gritting my teeth, trying to get my core muscles to knit together. I knew it was probably really inadvisable and I knew I was risking not healing properly, but there's no way I could have laid in bed for six weeks, except under sedation, and I didn't want that either.

I kept myself busy by catching up on all the outstanding admin, and I drifted in and out of naps, but most of my time was spent heaving myself out of bed and waddling to the toilet as fast as I could, often for the fourth time that hour, losing the will to live and hoping that I wasn't about to have another humiliating clean-up operation to deal with.

I eased myself slowly back into bed, and got myself into a tolerable position. I'd just opened my laptop and logged on to check my emails when my phone rang. It was Dad. He was outside, giving Bran and B their dinner.

'Alexis, it's B,' he said. 'She's collapsed.'

I could hear the panic in his voice. My stomach lurched as a surge of adrenaline hit.

'What? Right. I'm coming . . .' I braced myself and stood up. Barely noticing the pain it must have been causing, I made my way downstairs, through the house and out the back door. Using the fence to hold myself up, I staggered round to the hospice.

Through the darkness, in the glowing light from B's bedroom, I could see Dad crouched next to her with his hand on her side. B was lying on her side panting, trembling and barely conscious.

A few days before, five days after I got out of hospital, B had gone in for surgery to remove a small mammary tumour that had appeared. Her vet thought it was best to get it off sooner rather than later, given her history, and as she seemed to be in good health otherwise, she was a good candidate for surgery. She was an older lady, now, but her heart and lungs were strong, and her blood tests hadn't flagged up any problems with her liver, kidneys or anything else that might cause concern. It had been a fairly straightforward procedure, as these things go, especially compared to what she'd been through before. She'd been recovering in her bedroom, but Dad had said that morning that he didn't think she was feeling as well as she should be. The anaesthetic seemed to have really floored her. Dad had brought her to the gate and I'd inched my way through the mud to meet her and see what I thought. I agreed: she didn't look like herself. A tiredness had crept into her once-bright and keen eyes. She couldn't be bothered. Something was missing.

'What happened?' I said now, as I eased myself down, wincing as bits of regrowing tissue stretched and tore apart.

'I d-don't know,' stuttered Dad. He was pale, and shaken by the fright. 'She was like this when I came in. I went to get her dinner and . . .'

'How long has she been like this?' I reached for my phone. I'd forgotten to bring it out with me. *Shit.*

'I saw her a couple of hours ago. She was tired and a bit fed up, but she was OK. She definitely wasn't like this . . .'

'Right, OK, we need to get her to the car. She needs to get to the vet. I don't know what's wrong, but this isn't good.'

'Mnnnnmnnnnn,' I moaned. Every bump in the road sent a shockwave of pain through my guts.

I wasn't supposed to be out of bed for at least six weeks, and I wasn't supposed to be outside with the animals for twelve. Now I was in the back of the car, on my way to the vet, with a dog lying on my knee. I'd been home for six days.

As we made our way along the dark country roads, I could barely see B's shadowy outline against my clothes. I could hear her breathing, fast and shallow, and her nose and ears were raging with a fever. She seemed to be drifting in and out of consciousness, and every so often she'd moan, almost under her breath. B was rarely demonstrative. Aloof, independent, cheerful, and the only one of us who got any respect from Charles the dickhead turkey whose aggressive nature meant he usually went in on the attack, aye; demonstrative, no. I could have a walk-by kiss on the hand once a month and consider myself lucky.

I was in shock. I'd not been expecting this. I'd no idea what was happening, but I already knew I'd never see B again, not the whole B. Not the B-Bop-A-Loo-Bop-A-Woppa-Bamma-Boom-B – the affectionate, made-up, ridiculous nickname that I always called her by. I knew that the thing that had made her *her* was in the process of winding things up, here.

As gently as he could, Dad lifted B off my knee and carried her into the vet clinic. Behind him, I willed myself out of the back of the car and up the step to the door of the surgery. By the time I got in and lowered myself down into the plastic chair in the corner of the consulting room, B was lying on her side on the table and the vet was listening to her chest, looking concerned.

'Her heart's racing. She's crashing,' he said, taking off his stethoscope. 'I'm going to give her fluids and morphine. And some IV antibiotics, in case it's an infection. I don't know what's causing it, but we need to get her temperature down, fast.'

I looked at him, and down to B, lying on the table. She was barely conscious, and she looked like she was getting worse, not better. I half-stood up and shuffled my chair forward, reaching out for the tan sock on her front paw.

'What's happening?' I asked. 'Is it to do with the surgery?' It was the most obvious thing; it had been really hard on her. 'Or the cancer?' I was trying to work out what was going on, what we were preparing for, what might be about to happen.

'I don't know. Possibly. It could be an infection, or it could be the cancer has spread. We'll know more in the morning.'

'Is she staying in tonight?' I didn't want to leave her, but I knew she needed to be there.

'Aye, she'll need to stay here tonight, on the drip and the pain relief. It could be pain that's causing her fever. Really bad pain can do that.'

Pain so bad it makes you collapse, panting and groaning. That sounded familiar.

'I know, B-Bop. I know.' I squeezed her paw. 'Stay brave. I'll see you soon, OK?'

I straightened the duvet and shuffled around a bit, trying to get comfy. B was beside me, doing the same. She sighed, and rested her chin on her paws. I picked up my book and reached over to rest my hand on her back.

Overnight, her heart rate and breathing had started to get back to normal, and by morning, she was awake and alert. But we'd found our answer: something was blocking the normal flow of her lymphatic system, and, unable to drain, it had caused one of her back legs to swell up. There was no hiding the obvious culprit. The cancer was spreading, and it was travelling through her on her body's expressway.

The vet had asked me to take her home and keep her comfortable, and said that, if the swelling didn't rectify within forty-eight hours, it wasn't going to. And, if it didn't, I knew what B would decide.

I could barely stand up, myself; it took a lot of doing, but I collected a few duvets and blankets from around the place and made us two beds near each other on the living-room floor. B liked her space, and so did I, but side by side, we lay there, both cut open and stitched back up the middle, both feeling rotten, vulnerable and undignified. B didn't want to be lying there worried about humiliating herself in front of someone any more than I did.

'Mmmmggghhhhh,' I groaned.

'Mmmmmmmmmnnnggghh,' B responded, rolling over.

Aye. We each knew exactly what the other was going through.

B loved Ringliggate. On rounds, she'd come up the hill with me and go off to gather information for the next quadrant of her sniff map, rejoining me back down the hill at the gate, bouncing in anticipation of the breakfast waiting for her in her bedroom. I'd not had a lot of time, with everything else that had been going on, and I'd not had much energy for long walks lately, but we'd had a few days out to local beaches and down in Kirkcudbright, getting all the smells.

The cottage in Ballindalloch had been as stressful for her as it had been for the rest of us, and she was enjoying the peace – if living next door to a dog with a loudspeaker instead of a voice box can be described as 'peace' – and the independence she had in her new home. Given the choice, B would always choose to go off and do her own thing. I'd stopped letting her off her lead after she'd gone AWOL a few times up in Ballindalloch, away down the hill, through the woods, towards the river. One time she wandered off, she brought a cockerel home (it's a long story). She had been getting frustrated at not having her freedom, but now she was exploring the mysteries of Ringliggate and the new world around her with a spring in her step and a sparkle in her eyes that I'd not seen for far too long.

'How you feeling, B?' I started turning myself over. I'd drifted off, and it was getting dark.

B was lying still, but I couldn't tell in the gloom if she was sleeping.

'D'ye want to try some eggs, B-Bop? Give it a go, eh?'

I reached round and turned on the lamp. She was following me with her eyes, her tan eyebrows twitching and bobbing above them. She'd always had a good appetite, but she was finding fewer and fewer things appealing, and the only thing she was even remotely interested in now was scrambled egg.

'Right, I'll go and get it ready. D'you want to go outside, first?'

Back in the living room, I rearranged her duvets and blankets and helped her get settled. She was finding it difficult to move by herself, and if the swelling in her leg felt anything like that time when I thought I'd broken my foot, in Aviemore, then it must have really bloody hurt. I'd been massaging ginger oil into it, hoping that it might help alleviate some of the swelling, but it was getting worse, not better. Unlike Bran, who was quite happy to trample about in his own jobbies, knowing that it was someone else's problem, B was really upset at feeling her dignity slipping away.

I felt dreadful. My body was reeling from the shock of the operation, and the dust was still settling in my mind. But I was pushing on, and every day I felt a bit stronger, more resilient. I had a long way to go, and it would take months before I was fully mended, but I could feel my body starting to gather its strength. But B was going the other way. The swelling on her leg was spreading, now, further up her thigh and towards her hip. Hunger must have been starting to gnaw at her, and she was hurting from the shame and embarrassment of having to be nursed and cleaned. Every day, I was watching B grow weaker.

We'd held the cancer at bay for two and half years – two and a half years longer than we originally thought we'd be able to. B had staked her claim on life, but she was fading and this was only going to go one way.

My friend didn't want to fade away, didn't want to lose the dignity and independence that were so important to her. I wouldn't want that for myself and I didn't want that for her, either. It was almost forty-eight hours since Dad had carried B out of the vet clinic and brought her home. Taking a deep breath, I picked up my phone and called the vet.

Shifting and wincing, I tried to get comfortable. We had a couple of hours left. B was watching me, looking as fed up as I felt. Reaching over, I put my hand on her back.

'I know, B-Bop.' I smiled over to her.

She lifted her eyes to look at me for a moment, then let her gaze fall back to the floor.

I leaned over and kissed her head. 'I know.'

CHAPTER FIFTEEN

The Feral Jobby Trampler

'Right, Shitter McDitter, wait there . . . DON'T JUMP!'

As the pain-in-the-arse electric boot slowly groaned open, I crouched down with my arms spread, like I was defending a hockey net. The daft auld dog was likely to launch himself out of the car without thought for the consequences, but if I was quick enough, I'd be able to catch him mid-air.

'Brandon Fleming – patience! Wait a minute, till I get yer coat on . . .'

It was Valentine's Day, and despite it being grey, wet and about two degrees, I'd decided that Bran and I were going to have a Valentine's date, down at the beach. We were parked outside the small supermarket in Kirkcudbright, where I'd bought some ice cream and a bunch of flowers for our date, and I thought auld Shoogly might enjoy a wee potter round the streets before we went and got our chips and headed for the beach.

'Is that . . . Is that *Bran*?'

Startled, I looked round. A woman carrying laden shopping bags was peering, star-struck, into the boot.

'Hi, sorry, I'm Tracy,' she stammered. 'I follow your Facebook page. I hope you don't mind, I just cannae believe I'm actually meeting Bran in person!'

I laughed. 'Hey, Shoogly, you've been recognised, pal.'

'Do you think he would like a sweetie? I've always got some in my pocket . . .' asked Tracy, grinning and all but getting her autograph book out.

Bran's eyes weren't great, and he was (selectively) deaf, but there was nothing wrong with his nostrils and he knew a sweetie when he smelled one. Bran was homing in and he was just about in her pocket.

'Aye, I'm pretty sure he'd like a sweetie . . . Just mind yer fingers; he's like bloody Jaws!'

Leaving Bran in the car for a couple of minutes, I found a picnic spot on a little grassy outcrop at the top of the beach and unfolded the pretty embroidered tablecloth I'd bought at the charity shop for a few pennies, searching around for some stones to hold down the corners. We called this place 'Bran's Beach', and it was one of our favourite places. The high tide is very high, but at low tide, the flat expanse of sand reaches out into the bay towards the lighthouse – and beyond, over towards the Isle of Man. Today, I could barely see the distant water. It was a still day, but bitterly cold, and it really wasn't the weather for a picnic on the beach, but I knew we weren't going to get another Valentine's Day together, and we were used to making the most of – or, more accurately, working around – the Scottish weather. While I arranged our table, within easy distance of the car, I could hear the auld yin starting to lose patience.

'WOOF. WUMMIN.' *CHIPS!* 'WOOF! WOOF!'

'Aye, I hear ye! Gimme a minute, Branigan.'

He was pacing, fed up of waiting.

'Right, let's get some chips in us, eh Shitter?' I said, pressing the button to open the boot, and getting ready to catch.

He launched himself into my arms and I lowered him down as he doggy-paddled in mid-air, ready for action as soon as his big bear paws hit the ground. Sure enough, off he went, careering towards the bumpy outcrops, following his nose to the chips.

'Brandon, slow down!'

He had no sense of danger, and no regard that he was about 146 years old. Wrapped up against the cold, grinning like teenagers, we sat on our tablecloth and ate our chips and ice cream, taking some photos to share with his devoted online pals. One chip for me, four chips for Bran . . .

'Oi, mind my fingers, dickhead!'

'WUMMIN! WOOF! WOOF!' *CHIPS!* 'WOOF!' he shouted at the sky.

I scratched his neck and pulled him closer for a hug. 'Chips down the beach, pal. Doesnae get much better than this, does it?'

'Right, Branigan Shenanigan, let's get yer room ready . . .' Armed with a pile of folded laundry, I made my way through the hospice to his bedroom. Bran had always wobbled a bit on his ancient legs, but in the last few weeks, he'd been getting more unsteady on his feet. His old bones creaked and groaned, and my heart ached as I saw his already shoogly back legs get visibly weaker. It hadn't dented his will any, but there was no doubt that he was slowing down. There had been a couple of times when I'd had to carry him back to the car on walks that, not that long ago, he'd managed without thinking about it.

To prevent him from hurting himself with his slips and stumbles, I'd made his bedroom into one big bed, with thick piles of duvets, blankets and waterproof protectors covering the floor. For an auld man who loved his bed, he was pretty pleased with the my-whole-room-is-a-bed situation. Every inch of the floor was covered, and once it was done each night, I liked to stop for a moment and enjoy the fleeting pleasure of it being fresh and clean. By morning, I'd be considering napalm as a viable option for dealing with the shit show that it had become overnight. I've never met anyone who could create such utter devastation while they were supposed to be asleep. Nor had I ever met anyone who could decorate with jobbies quite the way Bran could. Living up to one of his many nicknames, the Feral Jobby Trampler would do his poo and then . . . Actually, I don't know how a twenty-year-old dog managed to get a big dollop of shit three inches from the ceiling.

'It's been a big day, eh, Shoogles? Beach, chips AND ice cream? You're so spoiled, y'know that?' I knelt down beside him on the rug and kissed the bony ridge on the top of his head. 'Come on, you, it's bedtime. Out for a wee.'

Slowly, he started to ease himself up, and I winced as his old bones creaked into action. I put my hand on his side to help steady him as he got his balance.

He enjoyed wandering about the field on his own, and lately I'd been keeping a close eye, just in case. As he sniffed and pottered, I leaned against the doorframe, yawning and blinking against the tiredness. He'd always been demanding, but as age took its toll, Bran needed and wanted more and more time and care, and he'd become a lot more persistent and impatient. I understood, but looking after him was two full-time jobs, with no days off, and I still had to fit in all the other jobs of the day. I was completely worn out.

'Right, you, come on. Bedtime.'

Satisfied that he'd got every last sniff, Bran started shoogling his way back to the hospice. His body was slowing down, but there was nothing wrong with his mind or his appetite, and it was time for the last sweeties of the day.

'Lucky dip, sir?'

As he padded around and turned in circles on his duvet to get it just right, I hauled myself through to the kitchen to get the lucky-dip bowl. Sometimes, we played catch for a while at bedtime, but I figured we'd had enough excitement for one day, and I really, really wanted my bed.

'WUMMIN!' *SWEETIES!* 'WUMMIN! WOOF! WOOF! WOOF! WOOF!'

'Aye, aye, I'm coming. Here ye go . . .'

I held the bowl of sweeties in front of him and tried to focus through my dry contact lenses.

'Look at ye, straight in there, no messin' . . .'

I laughed as he shoved his face in and rooted around for his favourites.

'Hey, Jaws, calm down!'

I took the bowl from under his nose and he dropped his haul on his bed in front of him.

'Five wee ones and a big one, is it? What is this, fecking *Countdown*, pal?'

By the time the nights were getting noticeably shorter and the world was starting to come back to life, we were all thoroughly fed up with winter. There was a lot of work still to be done outside, and as soon as funds permitted, I was going to get a car park, paths and hard standing done, and get rid of the mud once and for bloody all. There was still no running water, so even filling a mop bucket was a hassle – and the Feral Jobby Trampler suite alone often took at least two – as I carted another five-litre bottle of water from the house to the hospice.

'Fancy scrambled eggs for breakfast today, Shenanigan?'

Bran was watching me from a sunny spot on his rug, following me with his eyes as I got the mop ready to face the devastation in his bedroom. The most important thing about the hospice was always that it had to feel like home. As far as I could work out, Bran had never had a proper home of his own; he'd spent most of his life alone in a kennel. When we met, I promised him he'd have his own home one day, built just for him. Many times, it had seemed like an unachievable task. But the first time Bran shoogled out of his bedroom into his newly furnished living room and plonked himself down on the round grey rug in the middle of it, feeling like master of the universe, all the years of preparation, fundraising, building, disruption, worry and stress evaporated into distant memories. He'd waited a lifetime for it, but auld Shoogly finally had a home of his own, and he loved it.

Finally, an uplifting, promising warmth was blowing in on the breeze. All winter, I'd been hoping that we'd get one more spring and summer of walks and car trips and sunbathing together. We loved our days together in the sun.

'It's lovely out there today, Branflake. Might even be nice enough for a nap in the *car*! What d'ye reckon?'

CAR! 'WUMMIN! WOOF! WOOF!' *CAR!* 'WOOF! WOOF! WOOF! WOOF!'

'Aye, thought ye'd like that idea . . . Come on, then. I think it might be time to put on yer spring collar . . .'

I knelt beside him in his warm sunny spot on his rug and ran my hands over up over his face and down his neck, and kissed his nose. Eyes closed, he basked in the sun and the attention.

'I take it that feels good?' I laughed, as he did his happy-as-can-be lopsided grin and melted into the rug, groaning. 'Look at the state of ye, Shoogles. Ye sound like a drunk Chewbacca . . .'

A few months ago, Bran and I had arrived home late one evening. Doing my usual hockey-goalkeeper routine, I waited to catch him as he launched himself out of the boot, but as the boot lifted, I realised something was wrong. Confused and alarmed, Bran was swaying and tilting to the left, staggering sideways.

'Oh, shit, Bran – what is it, what's wrong?' Panic and fear surged through me as I tried to take in what was happening. Quickly, I scooped him up and lifted him out of the boot and on to the ground. He staggered, stumbling towards the wall, like a drunk trying to act sober at four a.m. *Shit, shit, shit.* It was late on a Sunday and I didn't want to disturb his vet without good reason, but this couldn't wait. My heart was pounding as I got my phone out of my pocket.

'It's OK, son, it's gaunnie be OK . . .' I didn't know if I was telling him the truth. What if it was time? What if he looked at me and knew? My stomach lurched. Looking for comfort, he burrowed his head into my chest, and I wrapped my arms around him. I could feel that he was worried, too.

His vet, Giselle, lived at the farm just up the hill, and she got to us within minutes. By torchlight, she watched him as he staggered and swayed around, his head low and twisted to the left. I could hardly bear to watch, and I was dreading what Giselle might be about to tell me. *Please, please, don't let it be time . . .*

'He's had a mini-stroke,' Giselle said as she stood up, removing her stethoscope.

'Is he gaunnie be OK?' Frantic, desperate, I crouched down beside Bran, who was already starting to look more aware and steady on his feet.

'Aye, I think so. It probably looks worse than it is. It's really common in older dogs; we see it all the time. There's a medicine he can take long term that will help. He'll be tired; the best thing for him now is plenty of sleep, and we'll see him again in the morning.'

I lifted Bran back into the boot as Giselle got his medicine ready and gave him a couple of injections. Overwhelmed by relief, feeling like we'd just rolled off the tracks as the train sped past, I thanked her, and waved as she set off, back up the hill.

Shaken, Bran and I sat side by side in the boot, taking in what had just happened. I could hear the burn that ran alongside the house, trickling and bubbling its way down to the sea, and a light breeze was moving the dry leaves still clinging to their branches. In the distance, a couple of tawny owls were having a conversation. A sob lurched up from my belly.

'Right, you, c'mere.' I turned to face him, and wrapped my arms around his neck.

Tired, he pressed himself into me, letting me take his weight. The medicine was working and he seemed to be through the worst of it, but it had really taken it out of him and the auld man was falling asleep sitting up.

As my shock started to wear off, the tears began to well. For a few moments, I'd thought I was about to lose my pal. I wasn't ready. I'd never be ready, but I knew I needed to do something I'd not had the courage to do before.

'Right, you, listen to me.' I steadied myself and, in the dim glow from the wee light in the boot, I looked into his face. 'I promise – promise – that, when you tell me it's time, I'll listen.' Holding his old, grey face in my hands, I kissed the cold velvety bit just above his nose. I felt another sob lurch up from the pit of my stomach. 'You promise to tell me, and I promise I'll listen. Deal?'

I didn't want to face the thought of life without Bran, and I didn't want to think about the moment that was bound to come. But what had just happened had shaken me to the core, and it had made me realise how unprepared I was. It would come for all of us, but Bran was nearing twenty years old and there was no holding back the tide of decay and age. The inevitable moment was going to come, no matter whether I wanted it to or not. I could feel my heart fracturing just at the thought of it, but I needed to be ready and to have the strength to do what I needed to do for my pal, when I needed to do it. I couldn't panic, or be afraid, or doubt what he was telling me. One day, he would tell me, and on that day, I'd listen. With almost unbearable anguish at accepting the inevitable, I'd done it – I'd made the unbreakable promise, set in stone.

As spring got going, it was fast approaching three years since Bran and I had met. His willpower and love for life were incredible.

'Three years, hey, Shoogles?'

He lifted his head from its resting place on his big clumsy paws, which were crossed over each other in front of him.

'I think you should have a party, Branigan. What d'ye think?'

We needed a celebration. He had so many pals online who adored him, but he'd never met most of them. While I did his Facebook posts every day and shared his stories and our conversations, it was easy to forget that, though I knew how much love there was out there for this smelly auld dog, he didn't even know these folk existed. I told him often enough how many people loved him, but it wasn't the same as feeling that love in person. And, being practical, as auld Shoogly got shooglier, if we were going to celebrate, it would have to be sooner rather than later.

I picked the weekend closest to his gotcha day – the day he arrived at the hospice, in 2017 – and within a few minutes, I had it all planned in my head.

Sunday 2 June 2019 was going to be Bran Day.

Straight away, I started putting invites up on Facebook. With only two weeks' notice, I wanted to make sure as many folk as possible could come. A lot of his further-away Bran fans wanted to join in, too, and over the next few days, as we organised the raffle, treasure island, barbecue and nightmarish parking and facilities logistics, parcels and messages started to flood in from around the world. Beautiful, thoughtful gifts addressed to the Feral Jobby Trampler, Shitter McDitter, Shoogly McDoogly, Bran the Man, SuperBran, Branigan Shenanigan and his many other nicknames gave the postie a laugh and swelled my heart.

A long-time supporter of the hospice, Nicola, offered to design some special Bran Day T-shirts for his fans, and another supporter offered to make him a cake. It was bone-shaped, peanut-butter flavoured and decorated with big bold letters: *Feral Jobby Trampler*.

There was still a lot of work to be done in the hospice. The three bedrooms were half-finished and needed to be painted and decorated, and a couple needed to be tiled, too. There was still no running water or toilet, and the kitchen was in bits, in what was eventually to become the wet room. The warmer weather had at least dried the mud out, and the hospice was functional enough to keep us warm and dry for the party, should the weather not be on our side. There was enough room for about twenty people to mingle and enjoy the cakes and treats that folk were sending as their contributions to Bran Day, and we'd arranged a gazebo for the barbecue area, too.

We woke to an atmospheric, misty Sunday morning. Toby, a photographer, had agreed to capture the day for us, and he was outside getting photos of the chicken, turkey, sheep and pig folk, while I hastily made *No Parking* signs for the neighbours' grass verge, and a couple of volunteers sorted out gazebo-related emergencies. Too excited and anxious to eat, I nibbled at some breakfast and went out to do the morning rounds in plenty of time, before everyone arrived.

'Morning, pal!'

Bleary eyed, Bran was just starting to come to as I opened his bedroom door. His face was still crumpled from sleep and his top lip was curled up over his tooth.

'Time to get up. It's yer big day!'

He was lying on his new duvet cover – patterned with colourful toy *CARS!* – and I helped him put on his Superman collar, his new coat and a tartan bow tie – all gifts from his fans around the world. For a few moments, I stopped and looked at him, overtaken by emotion.

Before he met me, Bran had spent his days alone in a kennel. He'd gone to bed alone and he'd woken up alone, longing for a kind hand to reach out to comfort him and ease his loneliness. I didn't know how long he'd been waiting there, but I knew he'd been lonely for a long time. His frantic need for – and reaction to – affection, when we first met, made it obvious that love and kindness were not the norm for Bran. When his old body had started to wear out, disease and cause bother, he'd been discarded on the street, with as much care and thought as a bin bag of rubbish. Had he hoped for the day when someone noticed him? How did his unloved heart and lonely soul keep going all those years, through the pain?

But now, the old, unloved, unwanted dog, who so nearly lived a whole lifetime without love lighting up his heart, was about to be celebrated with a party to rival the best of them. Sitting beside him on his duvet, snatching a few moments before folk started arriving and everything got into full swing, I planted kisses on his head and gave him a squeeze. I wiped a tear away with my sleeve.

'They're all coming here for you, son. Everyone has done this for you . . .'

The sky cleared as party time drew closer, and soon the guests began to arrive. Mum and Dad had brought along their latest foster dog, Kilo – a cheerful American bulldog lad, with a huge, untreated and inoperable tumour on his leg – and along with the other guests, they were chatting and enjoying the cake and snack buffet on the lawn.

Meanwhile, Bran and I were trying to contain our excitement, as we sat in the boot of the car, waiting for Dad to come and give the signal for the star of the show to make his grand entrance.

'That's us ready . . .' I said, watching as Dad opened the main gate and made his way to meet us.

As we went to greet the guests, Bran was in his element, basking in the love of the day. I'd been worried it would be too much for him, but I'd been worrying about the wrong person. It was me who was finding the whole thing too emotional and overwhelming.

'So many folk have come, Dad . . . They've all come to see Bran.'

'Aw, love, I know – it's all a bit much, isn't it? But it's good, though. I hope those are happy tears.' He put his arm round me and pulled me in for a hug.

'They are.' I sniffed, laughing at myself. 'It's just . . . he's so special.'

'Come on, this is a happy day.' He reached into his pocket and handed me a tissue. 'Look what Bran has done! So many people love him, and – look at him – he knows.'

I looked down at Bran, panting with excitement and beaming from ear to ear. Dad was right. Bran was so special, and today he was going to feel like the king of the world.

As willing as Bran was, his body wasn't a match for his determination, so as Toby captured the moment, I scooped Bran into my arms and carried him towards his waiting guests in the hospice. Dad walked beside me and as we opened the gate, our eyes met and he saw overwhelmed, overjoyed tears welling in my eyes again.

He shook his head, laughing. 'Come on, you big softie.'

Through the glass, I could see that the hospice was packed with eager faces anticipating the arrival of the main man. Bran fidgeted in my arms, impatience getting the better of him again.

'Right, son, here we go . . .' Nervous and excited, I braced myself as Dad opened the door, and we stepped inside.

'Happy Bran Day to you! Happy Bran Day to you! Happy Bran Day, dear Shoogly! Happy Bran Day to you! Hip hip, hooray!'

The hospice erupted in applause and laughter. In my arms, Bran looked from me to the crowd and back to me, as it began to dawn on him: *They're all here to see me . . .*

I lowered him to the ground. For a few moments, he stood motionless on his rug, taking in the scene. Slowly, he looked from person to person, and I could almost hear the cogs turning as he struggled to take it in. *They're all here . . . for me . . .*

'WOOF! WOOF! WOOF!'

'Aw, Shoogly, look at yer face!' I knelt down beside him for a wee reassuring cuddle. 'Come on, son, why don't you go and say hello to everyone?' I helped him shoogle over to his fans, and immediately he was lost in the fuss and attention, going from person to person, lapping it up.

'Look at his face – he's absolutely loving it!' Alan, the guy with the transport truck, who had helped us move into our new home during those eventful days the year before, was almost as emotional as me. 'I made you something,' he said, and he handed me a large rectangular package.

It was a painting of Bran that he had done for me.

'Oh, Alan, I love it! Thank you so much.' We hugged, and I was away again, tears flowing.

Once Bran had done his rounds, I gathered him up and settled him on a red blanket in front of his table of presents.

'Hey, Shitter, these are all for you, pal!'

He grinned up at me, his old eyes sparkling.

We opened a few presents and everyone watched, delighted, as he ripped and tore at wrapping paper, nosing from one parcel to the next, hardly believing his luck. For an old dog, who had waited a long time for anyone to notice him, he was absolutely relishing the attention. But he was getting tired, now; there was only so much excitement an ancient old man could handle.

'Right, auld yin, I think that's enough, for now. Time for a nap.'

As the party wound down and the clear-up operation began, the day and all it had meant started to catch up with me. As I shared photos online, I saw the messages folk had sent from around the world: Leonie in New Zealand; Judy in South Africa; Hendrika, Louis, Pam and Annabelle in the States; Bo in the Netherlands; and so many more. In an ever-dividing world, a shared love for this auld man had brought people together in celebration of what he'd achieved. Bran Day was a manifestation of the love for him that had started and spread in the online world, brought to life in the real one. For so long, he'd waited to be known and loved, and now he knew that he was.

In the quiet of the summer evening, I tucked a blanket around my auld pal's shoulders.

'I could curl up in there beside ye, Shoogly . . .' Yawning, I kissed his head and massaged my hands over his shoulders. He was absolutely exhausted, and ready for a good long sleep.

'Yer a very loved auld man, Brandon Fleming. Night night, sweetheart.' I kissed him again, turned out his light and, buoyant, walked back to the house.

*

'WOOF! WUMMIN! WOOF! WOOF! WOOF!'

'I'm coming, Bran, I'm coming . . .'

Up on the hill, I had almost finished the rounds. Bran had woken up from his nap in the car, and he was wondering where I was. Over the last few weeks, he'd become more dependent, and he didn't like to be alone for even a second. I'd started sleeping in the hospice, and the unsettled nights as he padded around in the dark were taking their toll. His back legs were getting weaker almost by the day, and though his medication was keeping him from being sore, he needed to be carried in and out of the hospice now, and more and more often, he needed help just staying upright on his ever-shorter potters around the field.

My hopes for one more summer together had come true, though, and we'd spent day after day lying on a duvet on the grass, soaking the heat of the sun into our aching bones. He loved the sun. Side by side, smiling, not doing much of anything except being together, we spent hours just enjoying each other's company. We were tired in different ways. I wasn't getting much sleep, and the demands of the sanctuary and my auld pal were sometimes stretching my patience to its limits.

'WOOF! WUMMIN! WOOF! WOOF! WOOF!'

I'd just sat down with a cup of tea, drained, worried, frustrated, exhausted. I couldn't handle any more, not today. I stormed over to his door.

'WHAT? *What* do you want, Bran? For fuck's sake, there's *nothing* else I can give you! Please . . . just fucking *stop!*'

Guilt tore at me as the words came out my mouth, and his confused old eyes looking up at me etched themselves forever on my heart and soul. I was all he had, the only person he had to rely on, and I'd scared him. I couldn't bear it. I was utterly exhausted, but it wasn't an excuse. I crumpled on the floor beside him, sobbing, kissing him, reassuring him, telling him how sorry I was and promising I'd never lose my temper with him again. My tears fell on to his fur, and he kissed my nose. *It's OK, wummin. It's OK.*

Walks were becoming more difficult, but he was still raring to go, so over summer, we started taking long drives in the car. I'd put a duvet on the front seat and buckle him in. Lost in joy, we'd twist and turn along the country roads, music blaring, windows down, Bran with his lopsided happiest-of-happy grins.

'You're the song in my heart! You're the song in my hea-rt . . .' I sang, badly, as loud as I could. 'That's you, pal!' I smiled down, tickling his neck.

As August rolled round, we were starting to take things even slower. In the hospice, I'd moved from the sofa bed to the floor, moving his my-whole-bedroom-is-a-bed set-up to the living room, so that we could sleep beside each other. He was still loving his sweeties, and I'd no idea how a dog who was more than twenty years old could still be such a master at a game of catch, but he'd started to become fussy about his home-made dinners and I was having to tempt him more and more often with cheap, tinned food for his regular meals, because that, apart from scrambled egg (and the aforementioned sweeties), was the only thing left that he'd eat.

I knew what was coming. My shoogly auld pal knew, too. It wasn't quite time yet, but I was preparing myself for the day he told me it was. Every day, a thick grey cloud hung over me, waiting to unleash its pain and grief in a torrent.

'No dinner tonight, son? OK, how about a sweetie instead?' I offered him the lucky-dip bowl.

He had a disinterested sniff and turned away.

My heart was dipping in and out of grief with every rejected or eaten meal. 'I love you, auld man,' I told him. 'I love you so, so much . . .' Tears and snot flowed on to his fur. On the floor of the hospice, in the half-light at the end of a clear August day, we lay together on our thick pile of duvets. As I held his old, frail body close, the dread of the promise made all those months ago echoed through me. He was going to tell me, soon, and though it was the last thing in the world I wanted to hear, inevitability and time were knocking on the door, and there was nowhere to hide.

It was just after seven a.m. and a shard of bright, early morning sunlight cutting across the floor woke us from our restless night. Bran had been finding the nights harder as his pain medication struggled to keep up with his aches, and his old brain started to struggle to make sense of things that, not so long ago, he'd found comforting. He'd paced and panted through the night, and for the first time I'd seen him distressed by his old body. As I turned round to face him, I already knew.

Weary, he lifted his head, and our eyes met.

It's time, wummin.

My head dropped and I closed my eyes. Somehow, from somewhere, I had to find the strength I needed. Breathing through the sorrow that was flowing up from deep inside, I took a deep breath. I was lost in the place between life and death. *You made a promise. He trusts you. You have to do this.* I wrapped my arms around him and squeezed reassurance into him.

'It's OK, son. It's gaunnie be OK . . . We're gaunnie be OK . . .'

I kissed his head and tucked the duvet round his shoulders. Slowly, I stood up and went to the kitchen to prepare his breakfast. I hoped that some scrambled egg might tempt him to eat something before the vet came. A sob lurched up; I didn't want him to die hungry.

I was right – scrambled egg was just the ticket. He wolfed it down, and looked for more.

'Bloody typical, Brandon Fleming! Right, wait here – I'll make some more.' Smiling, relieved, I rubbed my hands through his glossy black fur. For such an auld stoater, he'd really kept his good looks.

Before I phoned the vet, I still had the rounds to do. I had no option; no matter what else was happening, there was always something that needed doing. Lost in thought, I quickly opened the huts, distributed food and refilled water dishes. The sun was warm on my face, but a cold dread was shivering through my bones. Time was ticking on. I took my phone from my pocket: 8.31. The vet clinic would be open now. *Fuck.*

I had a job to do, a responsibility to uphold and a promise to keep. Now wasn't the time for my cowardice. Without hesitating, I dialled the number.

'Hi – it's Alexis, up at the hospice. It's . . . it's Bran.' I held my voice steady. 'It's time . . .'

Bran and I had shared three and a half joyous, blessed, love-filled years together. There were so many upsetting, distressing, lonely or painful ways my ancient auld pal could have died that were outside my control, but he'd dodged them all. In the next couple of hours, I had the chance to make his death as good as the last few years of his life had been. It was our final blessing.

Carefully, I carried Bran out of the hospice to the car.

'How d'ye fancy a wee date down at the beach, Shoogly?' We had time for one more trip to our favourite place.

'WOOF! WOOF!' *CAR!* 'WUMMIN! WOOF!' *BEACH!* 'WOOF!'

'Aye, there's nothing wrong with yer voice box, is there, Shitter McDitter?' I made sure we had some of his favourite sweeties, and climbed in the driver's seat. 'Right, pal, here we go! One last song, for good measure. What d'ye say?'

I cranked up the music and, as we drove together to our special place for the last time, through tears of pure joy and crushing sorrow, I sang loud enough for even auld deafy to hear.

'You're the song in my heart! You're the song in my hea-rt . . .'

Just after ten thirty a.m. on Saturday 10 August 2019, in his car, eating his sweeties and wrapped in the arms of his wummin, with dignity, peace and love, Bran fell asleep and gently left behind his creaky, worn-out auld body, to take the path I couldn't follow.

Slowly, I walked to the house. Relief washed over me. My shoogly auld pal had had the perfect death, and now nothing could take those beautiful final moments away from us. No more worries, no more fear, no more aches or pains or what ifs. He'd never die alone or in pain. He'd never know anything other than peacefully slipping away, having his head massaged and his nose kissed and being told how much his wummin loved him. My shoogly auld pal had had exactly the death I wanted for him. He'd finally known gentleness and peace, in life and in death. He'd told me and I'd listened, and together, as we faced the unknown, we were given our last gift.

I opened the bottle of gin and poured some into a glass.

'Here's to you, Shoogly . . .'

I braced myself, downed the gin, put on my wellies, and went to clean the chicken sheds.

CHAPTER SIXTEEN

Keep Going

Even with Bran gone, there was no time to dwell on my grief. The wheel kept turning, life went on and there was always another animal pal who needed my help.

A few weeks before Bran left us, K had come to live at the hospice. She had been through a lot: her person had died, so she'd been taken to a kennel in a rescue centre; she'd been rehomed a few times, but none of the homes had worked out. When she'd started limping on one of her back legs, the rescue had some tests done, which showed what looked like a cancerous mass in her hip joint. Her prognosis was poor and the vet thought she might only have a couple of weeks left to live. The volunteers at the kennels were really fond of her, but she was highly excited by other dogs and being in a kennel was just way too stressful for her. They got in touch to ask if there was room for one more at the hospice, so that she could spend her final few weeks in a home, hopefully with some of the peace that had been missing from her life so far.

She arrived a couple of days later, and, fuelled by the stress, her natural Staffie exuberance was dialled up to bouncing-off-the-walls twenty-four seven. For a few weeks, I had to sedate her and sit with her, reassuring her, to get her to calm down enough for even a few minutes of restless sleep. But something wasn't adding up. There was a big difference between what I expected to see from a dog with end-stage cancer and the ginger blur with so much energy she didn't know what to do with it. She didn't seem to be in pain, and she certainly didn't seem to be in the last stages of her life.

I took her to my local vet for his opinion. He looked at her X-rays and he examined her, and then he said, 'This dog doesnae have cancer.'

It turned out that she had an old hip injury or disease, or possibly a birth defect, that had left her with a deformed hip joint and one leg slightly shorter than the other. Her bad leg was a bit weaker than her good one, and it got a bit sore if she really overdid things, but otherwise it really didn't bother her much.

As the months passed and we got to know, trust and love each other, K started to calm down and finally find the peace she'd been missing. These days, she was still bouncing off the walls, but it was fun bouncing, not frantic bouncing. I was delighted that she wasn't dying, but it meant I had a difficult decision to make. The hospice was for terminally ill animals, and K wasn't terminally ill, or even ill at all. But, as my heart had taken a battering as my shoogly auld pal faded away, K was blossoming and had filled me back up with her endless Staffie love. She was made to love and to be loved, and her huge smile and soft, content eyes got right into my soul. She needed someone, I needed someone, and we'd found each other. K and I decided that she was home.

She still liked to keep me on my toes.

'Right, you, walk time. Sit still till I get yer coat on . . .'

K threw herself at the gate of her outside run and turned in circles as I manhandled her into her coat and harness.

'Eeewwwaaaeemmmaaargh!'

K had a noise for every occasion, and none of them sounded like the noises dogs were supposed to make. With her finally in her coat and harness, and her lead wrapped tightly around my wrist, I opened the gate. A walk with K was a no-messing sort of affair. It was more like a drag – as fast as she could go, and in a straight line. It didn't matter where we were going, as long as we got there by the most direct route, as quickly as we could. A few weeks before, her attempt at proving herself to be the world's strongest dog, down at Bran's Beach, had ended in me rupturing the ligaments in my left ankle – I was hobbling for days – and our 'walks' up in the woods above Kirkcudbright were an assault course of fallen trees, trip-hazard roots, muddy puddles and undergrowth, all of which I was hauled over, under or through on the end of a leash attached to the wee ginger liability.

This afternoon, we walked up to the top of the hill across the road. I took in the view across the water, to the hazy outline of the Isle of Man, while K vibrated at the cows and made the kind of noise that I imagine a seal would make if it got stuck in a pipe.

I braced myself against a chilly south-westerly gust and tucked in my neck warmer.

'Ooof, K, that blows the cobwebs away, eh, doll?'

On our walks, we often stopped for a blether and shared passing waves with the people we bumped into. On our way back today, Stuart, the shepherd, stopped for a chat as he went about his rounds.

'Afternoon, Stuart. Hey, Rab.'

Behind him, Stuart's Border collie, Rab, sat poised and focused, raising a dignified and unamused eyebrow at the straining, wriggling, screeching ginger embarrassment-to-their-kind, which was making noises that he was pretty sure dogs shouldn't make.

'Cold one today, eh?' Stuart shouted over the racket.

Back in the warmth of the hospice, I got on with the cleaning and K went from toy to toy, wondering what to play with next.

'Where's your toys, K? Get them!'

She grinned her big Staffie grin at me, and grabbed the nearest toy proudly.

Mopping done, I plonked myself down on the sofa for a quick recharge with a cup of tea and a crossword.

'Oi, hyper, c'mere and give me a cuddle.'

Panting with excitement, she jumped up beside me, and I got my cup of tea out the way just in time.

'K, careful! Right, c'mere, you . . . Gimme that belly . . .'

As I rubbed and scratched her tummy, she writhed and wriggled and whirled on her back, kicking her hind legs and giving me sloppy kisses all over my face and hands, all the while continuing to practise her impressions of sea creatures stuck in drainage equipment.

I finished my tea and wandered over to the kitchen to fill her Kong with peanut butter for her evening's entertainment.

'Right, you, bedtime.'

She looked up at me, not wanting to go to her bedroom.

'Here you go, darling girl. Enjoy . . .' I handed her the Kong.

She hopped into her bed and now it was the Kong's turn for her undivided attention.

'See you later, sweetheart. I love you!' I don't think she even noticed me kissing her goodnight.

I closed her door and put the two twenty-kilogram weights in front of it. I loved my wee mental ginger dolly-bird angel to the stars, but I was under no illusions.

A few weeks later, K was joined by another new resident. Baggins (Billy when he arrived) had had a horrible life. A Great Dane cross, he had probably been taken on as a tough-looking 'status' dog, but his owner ended up in prison, so the guy's girlfriend was supposed to be taking care of Billy. He was found by chance in her back garden, starving and half-dead from an E. coli infection, with no bed and nothing but a sheet of plywood for shelter. He'd been neglected and slowly dying for at least two years. When Caz – the lady who found him – met Billy, she could fit her hands around his waist. It had taken her ten months to bring him back from the brink. She'd had to build him back up slowly, protecting his organs, which were dangerously close to failing, and treating his infections and wounds, and she spent months cleaning up the sprays of diarrhoea from the walls of her house as his broken body fought to survive.

Caz and I knew each other through Pounds for Poundies, and though she loved Billy deeply, as he started to heal, she realised he would be happier living out his final days at the hospice, where he could spend time outdoors, in a peaceful place, away from the city. Since Bran had died, the Feral Jobby Trampler suite was waiting to welcome its next charge, and so, on a wet, foggy night at the end of September 2019, Baggins came to join the party.

He still had a way to go, when he arrived. Caz had worked wonders for him, but his black fur was still dry and full of dandruff, and he just didn't have that spark that comes when the healing works its way from the inside to show itself on the outside. It took a while, but eventually his shine returned, and with it the long-suppressed inner puppy in his old eyes.

His body still bore the marks of his past, and he'd recently been diagnosed with degenerative myelopathy, which is a bit like a dog form of MS. He was slowly losing the use of his back legs. I gave him physio and plant medicines to keep him as healthy as possible, and he had a harness I used to help support him on his more difficult days, but eventually it started to become obvious that it was time for him to get some wheels.

The wheels came in the form of a set of stabilisers that fastened around his middle to help steady him. I was fairly certain he'd take to them without much upset; like Bran, not much bothered

Baggins, and he worked on the assumption that it was very charitable of him to give me something to do with my time. I was right, and within days he was a mobile menace, as he realised that his new wheels meant he could whizz round the place at lightning speed.

'Hey, Baggins?'

Whit?

'I'm just making a wee list, here, of all the things ye've stolen and run away with today. I've got a bag of apples, an empty packet of sweeties, a brown paper bag, a box of cat treats, a packet of herbal tea, a cardboard folder, a dog coat that's five sizes too wee for ye, a punnet of strawberries and a tin of coffee. Have I missed anything?'

Aye, add a cuddly toy and we'll be playing the fecking Generation Game, *wummin . . .*

I scanned the hillside as I battled with the padlock on the main gate. I'd only been out of the house for a couple of minutes and my hands were already frozen. I was always a bit tense when I first went out; much as I tried to keep everyone safe, I'd learned there would be days when I found someone was sick or injured on my rounds, or worse. Whether because I'd missed or forgotten something, or done something stupid or irresponsible, or because something unexpected, unforeseen and unavoidable had happened, some days went awry, and I'd learned that death doesn't always knock before stepping over the threshold. I'd come to accept that a constant background of mammy's worry just goes with the territory.

The sheep and a few of the cockerel bachelors were milling around among the gorse that was just starting to come out in its wee yellow flowers that made the place smell like suntan lotion. Some of the lads were having a meeting at the hang-oot tree – the distinctive sheltered gorse, silhouetted against the big sky, at the top of the hill. I did a quick sheep headcount. I had seven, now, and they were all present and correct. *Phew.* The Wee Yin, a black-face ewe with mischief shining out of her and horns that made her look like she had pigtails, was enjoying her morning butt-scratch against a gnarly old bush.

'Meh heh heh heh heh,' shouted Figgy from her sheltered spot up on the hillside.

'Morning, Fig. You OK, darlin?'

'Meh heh heh.' She was a fair-weather sheep, who hated getting mud on her dainty white feet, and like the rest of us, she was fed up with the wind and rain.

'Breakfast time soon, doll,' I shouted up.

It had been a dreich few days, a typical cold, wet and windy November, and today looked like it was going to be the same. It was bitterly cold, probably the coldest morning of winter so far. It had taken all my willpower to drag myself out of my bed in the dark. From the depths of my duvet, with my feet tucked into Ri's warm Staffie belly, the rain splattering against the windows of my bedroom was comforting and cosy, but it was a whole lot less comfortable and cosy being out in it.

The wee birds looked about as impressed with the weather as I was, and they darted around, blethering and commiserating with each other as they did their morning errands, while the jackdaws were making the most of it and having some fun in the wind. Next door, on the farm, the guys and their tractors had been busy since before dawn.

The pigs were already out of bed and up in their winter paddock, busy snouting around for roots and whatever else is worth spending hours searching for in the mud. I couldn't see the appeal, personally, but they assured me it was a great way to spend a morning.

A white cockerel was buk-buking around outside, waiting for me.

'Adam Jones! Hey, pal, how are ye doing today?'

Most mornings, we had a cuddle and a blether on our way up to Gimli and Elisa's paddock.

'This bloody mud, Adam Jones. This *bloody mud*!'

The work to the hospice and the land was still ongoing. The automatic water troughs and shed upgrades – courtesy of handyman Dad, as he muttered, 'Funny bloody retirement, this' – had helped make my daily tasks so much easier, and the new paths and car park that had been put in earlier in the year had been life-changing. The walk up to Gimli's field used to be a quagmire that I slipped, squelched and cursed my way through every morning, making it feel like I was doing daily training for a Tough Mudder. Glad to help once again, Dick, the local farmer, had stepped in and donated all of the rock for the paths from his quarry, saving the charity a small fortune in the process.

'MaaahhhhAAAAAAHH!' shouted Gimli across the field. He had an unusually squeaky voice for such a big sheep.

'Morning, Gimbolina!'

I worried more and more about Gimli. As time had gone on, his disability from his twisted spine and displaced hip had become harder and harder for him, and although he enjoyed life, I knew, without something to help support him, eventually it would become too much for him, physically and/or mentally. I really wanted him to have his freedom back and to be able to walk around without the strain, to be able to run around doing his excited zoomies that he loved so much. A prototype wheelchair someone very kindly made for him had proved to be too unstable. Desperate to help him, I was in the process of coming up with another plan – putting a zip wire in his paddock, along with a sling imported from the States. I was desperately hoping that my attempt at building a Go Ape for sheep might be the solution that worked for him, and I was determined to do everything I could to help him live his best life.

'MaaaaaaahAAAAAAAAH!' he shouted – not as patiently, this time.

'Aye, all right, Gimli. Gimme a minute, pal!'

Satisfied and relieved that everyone up on the hill was OK, I unlocked the door of the hospice and started to peel off my waterproofs.

'Morning, K! Morning, Baggins!'

I could hear them starting to stir in their bedrooms. The living room at the hospice was now taken up with our two newest guests – Badger and Digger.

The auld stoaters, as I called them, arrived at the beginning of September 2020. They were seventeen years old and I was told that they were brothers, but they were very strange-looking brothers. Badger was a cheerful wee Jack Russell fella, black and white, with an almost peach blush to his cheeks and an auld-man grey to his face. Diggity Dog was a grumpy, half-deaf, half-blind, more-fatty-lump-than-dog scruffbag of a cairn terrier. Their person, an old man who adored them, had died in the summer; although his family were really fond of Badger and Digger, they had other dogs, so they couldn't keep the two old men, and the hospice seemed like the perfect place for them to spend however long they had left. Their first few weeks here had been really difficult for all of us; they'd been through a lot and it was all really confusing for them. But – with some perseverance, routine, and lots of kisses and cuddles – slowly we were getting there.

'Morning, boys. Ewwww, what have you two been up to? It smells like an auld-man dog toilet in here . . .'

Curled up in his wee bed on top of a bigger bed, Badger startled awake and looked at me, blinking as the cogs behind his old eyes started to warm up. Digger was still out cold, stretched out on the thick memory-foam mattress in front of the heater. Badger peeled himself out of bed and tottered over to me, doing his morning stretches as I pulled down my waterproof trousers and took off my wellies.

'Oooooo, stretch it out, son. It feels goooood . . .' I bopped him on his shiny button nose as he stretched his paws out towards me and playfully gnawed at my hand. 'C'mere, you – give me a cuddle!' I picked him up, wrapped my arms around him in a big bear hug and smacked kissed all over his face.

Totally ignoring me, Badger was more interested in the cock pheasant rooting around in the vegetable patch outside the window.

'Come on, you – out of bed.' I knelt down beside Digger and brushed the hair out of his eyes as he started to wake up. 'Look at the state of ye, scruffbag.' I kissed his nose and wrapped my arms around him. 'Love love love yoooou,' I sang, as I squeezed him and tickled my way down his back.

Fully charged, he sprang out of bed and made for the door.

Badger tended to think that bouncing at the door might open it, while Diggity liked to try barking, to see how that worked.

'Wait . . . It's cold out there, this morning. Yer not going out without yer coats on . . .'

Holding them still, I fastened their winter coats around them.

'Right, you pair, out for yer wees.' I opened the door and the two auld men bounced out and ran off to start their day's adventures.

While they were seeing what the morning's sniffs had to offer, I set about clearing up the mess they'd caused while they were supposed to be sleeping. I began by checking how far they'd managed to pee under the fridge during the night. *Quite far*, was the answer. I cleaned up a bit and made their breakfasts, scattering a few treats around their beds for them to find on their sweetie treasure hunt when they got in.

Once they'd been out pottering for a while, I went to see if Digs needed help finding the front door again. 'Right, young men, in ye come,' I called. 'Breakfast's ready.'

Badger came running towards the door and took a flying leap up the step and into the living room.

'Aw, Badge, look at yer face! Ye excited, son?'

Digs, having found his own way back to the door, immediately started sniffing around inside, looking for the hidden treats.

'C'mere, coats off . . .' After freeing them from their coats, I knelt down beside Digs with his bowl. He sometimes needed a bit of encouragement to eat his breakfast – encouragement that, funnily enough, didn't seem to be necessary when it came to sweeties.

Pees and poos done, breakfast finished, treasure hunt complete, and the place smelling a bit less like auld-man dogs, it was time for a snooze.

There was certainly never a dull or a quiet moment, although sometimes it felt relentless – turkey and chicken sheds to clean, pigs and sheep to feed – but I loved having a catch-up with each of my pals. Whether it was a sheep, a cat or a bird, they each had their own distinct personalities. Take the turkeys: Angela, who hated getting out of bed in the mornings; her sister, Amber, who was constantly starting fights with the cockerels; and Charles, the dickhead turkey, who existed with the sole purpose of making my days as full of rage and as likely to end in injury as possible. When he wasn't threatening me with his free eyeball-removal service, he was barricading me in the chicken shed and threatening me with GBH if I tried to get out. This morning, he was perched on top of the nesting boxes.

'Got yerself stuck again, have ye, pal?'

'Bee bee doo boo. Beee boop be dooo boo.'

It was astonishing how he could make such sweet little noises sound like they were coming from the Kraken.

'Yer stuck and want me to help ye down? For real?'

'Boop beee doop BE DOOP BOO,' he replied, as he made a lunge for my skull.

'Right, come on then, ye prick. Yer something else, Charles, ye really are.'

I've never disliked someone in quite the same way as I disliked Charles, but I guess every family needs its token dickhead.

'Hilary, out of there!'

She'd made a beeline for the bag of sunflower seeds in the food shed, and she was in it head first, bum sticking out. She was one of the oldest ladies here now, but age hadn't dulled her sass any. She bullied her way to the front of the queue every morning, to get out the door first, so she could race to the food shed and get first dibs on what to shove her beak into. She'd got everyone wrapped round her little toe, and after she'd put most of the younger hens in their place, they'd quickly learned not to even bother arguing with her.

The hospice had recently expanded and we now had our very own cat wing. Its first residents – Archie and Josh – were curled up in bed together, in their shed. Until a few months ago, they'd lived on a landfill site; Mum had spent weeks trapping them and the other cats that were living there. She'd got them all neutered and had found most of them new homes for their much-needed fresh starts, but Josh had a long-term illness that made him difficult to home. He had nowhere to go, so Mum and I combined forces and built a big covered outdoor area for him to live in, at the bottom of the sheep field. Archie was healthy, but as Josh's devoted brother (or dad or cousin or uncle), he had to come, too. They mostly ventured out at night, and although Josh's eyes still had the look of a slow loris caught in headlights, I'd noticed that, in the last few weeks, there was a softness starting to creep in, and a couple of days ago, I'd seen them in daylight for the first time. We were not quite at the belly-rub stage yet, but we were heading in the right direction.

'Wean? Wean?' I shouted over to a lone jackdaw sitting on a post.

A few months ago, in late spring, a baby jackdaw had arrived. He'd fallen out of his nest in a local workshop, and there was nowhere else for him to go, so I became his mammy. He'd wake up and scream for his food every two hours, his huge yellow beak gaping open as a target. He liked cat food, blueberries and mealworms, and when he was really little and doing all his growing, he'd fall asleep almost the second he had finished eating. He was very dependent at first, and before he could fly, he sat on my shoulder while I did the rounds, watching and learning about the world.

Eventually, he started to find his wings, wanting to take the next step towards his independence, and he moved from his wee crate in the hospice into one of the isolation pens in the chicken field. I'd never known a jackdaw before, and getting to know the

Wean was a brilliant experience. He was my boy; I was his mum. At the end of every long summer day, just before bedtime, he'd be sitting on the same spot on his rope, waiting for me. He'd hop up on to my hand and we'd spend half an hour chatting to each other in little squeaks and clicks, rubbing our heads together, and he'd comb my hair with his beak.

I knew, one day, the wild in his blood would wake up and he'd have to leave, and I had been dreading it. One normal Sunday, a few weeks ago, he'd had his cat treat in the morning, sitting on my shoulder, and then hopped off to eat his breakfast. When I went back, later that afternoon, to give him his lunch, he was gone. It was a different sort of heartache, and it cut really deep.

I hope my Wean is up there, soaring and thinking he's the king of the world. I kept shouting for him, hoping that one day, he'd sneak away from his pals for a few minutes to let his auld mammy know he was doing OK.

'Wean?'

The jackdaw flew off. I smiled. It wasn't my pal. Not today.

First breakfast finished, Gimli had made his way over to his hay-rack for seconds.

'Look at yer face, Gimli. Have I ever told ye that yer the most handsome sheep in the whole world?'

He looked at me, his big lugs sticking straight up. He looked like a sheep, a llama and a kangaroo all rolled into one.

'Right, I've got to get going. I'll see ye later. Have a nice day!'

Hay under one arm and a bucket in each hand, I set off up the hill to feed the other sheep and to see to the bachelor lads. Adam Jones and his pals Alan Watts and Lord Flashheart followed along, buk-buking behind me.

'Ooo, what ye got for me today, Wattsicle?'

Alan Watts liked to bring me presents – little bits of flower or twig or sheep poo.

'Ooo, it's a bit of a leaf! That's lovely, pal.'

I discreetly put it back on the ground behind me, much like Mum used to do with the pinecones I collected for her and insisted she keep forever, when I was a kid.

Hazel, Figgy's sister and a food-obsessed mud magnet of a sheep, was licking her lips in anticipation of breakfast, careering towards the feeding trough and scattering cockerels like a woolly bowling ball. I barged my way through the throng of sheep and emptied the bucket into the trough.

While the sheep were distracted, I quickly heaved the bucket of the pig food up the hill. I was beginning to flag. A chilly draught was getting into my neck and my legs were starting to feel the strain as the last bit of energy from my morning's porridge was used up. My elbows were aching, my nose was running, and the ankle that K did a number on a few weeks ago was still causing a bit of gyp. *Urgh.*

'Come on, piggers, breakfast time! Ems, ye OK, doll?'

She heaved herself over to the fence for our morning blether, and so I could clean the mud off her eyelashes. 'Ooof ooof?' she asked.

'Oooof ooof.' I'd no idea what I was saying to her, but it seemed to satisfy her. She jogged off to join the others for breakfast.

'Brian, ye coming for breakfast, son?' A pair of lugs and a very sleepy face appeared at the entrance of their ark.

Brian never had any idea what was going on.

'Ach, son, I know how ye feel. Come and get yer breakfast – there's cabbage and pears today . . .' I scattered their breakfast on the rocky outcrop and left them to hours of digging and snuffling entertainment.

Up on his post, Jimmy Four Fingers, a local rook with a distinctive missing wing feather, was waiting for me to leave so he could swoop down and help himself to the pigs' breakfast.

I latched the gate and turned around for a lean, enjoying watching everyone tucking into breakfast, and enjoying that it was done and I didn't have to do it anymore, at least not for the next few hours. Bean, aka Major Douche, a magnificent goat with an attitude problem and an odd-couple living arrangement with a cockerel/lawsuit-waiting-to-happen called Rio, was tucking into his breakfast at his hayrack. Wanda – the newest sheep lassie to join us, who rivalled Hazel in the greed department and had a voice that made her sound like she smoked forty a day – was helping him from the other side of the fence, whether he wanted to share or not.

In the distance, I could hear the tractors at work in Dick's fields, and I don't know how the starlings lined up on the electricity wires could make out a word, the way they were chattering over each other. Down the hill, Baggins was out for his morning potter in his wheels, and he'd started shouting a demand of some sort. He'd either gone off-roading down the side of the hospice and got a wheel stuck on the downpipe again, or he was doing the exact opposite of what I'd asked him to do and was harassing the quail. Either way, I was going to have to go and resolve the situation he'd got himself into.

After I had dislodged Baggins from the downpipe, we made our way round to his bedroom.

'Right, Baggins, time to go in. Let's get ye out of those wheels . . .'

With Baggins settled, I hosed down his wheels, along with my wellies and waterproofs, and peeled off my mucky disposable gloves, looking around at everyone getting on with their day. Over in the chicken field, judging by the noise coming from one of the sheds, someone thought that the world was going to be as excited as she was that she'd just laid an egg, and there was some sort of turkey drama going on. I can feed, clean and nurse, but unless someone is going to lose an eye or suffer some other injury, I apply the same rule to chicken politics as I do to human politics: stay out of it.

My enthusiasm varies from morning to morning, and some-times my knees hurt, or my elbows ache, or my guts play up, or I'm in a grump. The last thing I want to do is go out and spend five hours in the rain. On those days, I could quite cheerfully stand out the front with a sign and throw the keys and the responsibility to the next unfortunate person who passes. Equally, there are those days when I know I'm the luckiest person in the world, because I've found the thing that gets me out of bed every morning just because I love doing it so much.

It can all feel a bit relentless sometimes, but no matter how sore or tired or unenthusiastic I might start out, the feeling, once everyone is happy and sorted and has everything they need for a safe and contented day, is always the same. Good days or bad days, they all make up the whole, and that whole is contentment. There's never been a day when I've not felt a bit better, even if it's just the simple satisfaction of having kicked myself up the arse and done it.

I turned the key in the hospice door and Badger blinked awake.

'Hey, Badge. Ooo, it's nice and warm in here. Get that kettle on, son – I'm ready for a cuppa . . .'

CHAPTER SEVENTEEN

The Black Cat

'Dad? What are you doing here?'

I pulled off my headphones and quickly dried my hands. Dad was standing in the doorway of the hospice, looking worried. I was standing in the kitchen, looking confused.

'You sounded a bit down, last night. I thought you could do with a hug.'

Dad and I talk every night, and he'd got a sense that I was starting to fray a bit round the edges. He was right: I had been struggling. Overtiredness always makes the normal day-to-day stuff a lot harder and more frustrating to cope with, so even the basics were feeling like they were a bit much. Months – years – of careering from a high to a low and back again, with not much time to process it all, was taking its toll, and I was starting to feel like I was permanently dialled up to twelve. The sense to get enough sleep and make proper meals, like a normal grown-up, often seemed to desert me, almost always trumped by my tendency to eat crisps for dinner and stay up till three a.m. going down Internet rabbit holes. A few other folk have vied for the title, over the years, but I really am my own worst enemy.

Emotionally, it had been a rough few weeks, too. As well as there being a few folk on palliative care to worry about, a couple of my pals had recently died within hours of each other. Chicken lass Bree faded away slowly over a few days as the dreaded ovarian-cancer time bomb went off and quickly spread its shrapnel through her body. I brought her into the house and nursed her, made sure she was warm, not sore, and I helped her sup her special nutritional drink. Like I had with Georgia, I knew her death was coming and that it was just a matter of time before she reached the expiry date she'd been born with. Late one evening, tucked in bed beside me, Bree's breathing slowed, her heart stopped, and she left very peacefully in her sleep. The next day, I buried her in the field where she'd spent her life.

A few hours after I'd said my final goodbye to Bree, Danny Carey, a young cockerel lad I'd known since he was a couple of days old, died very suddenly. It could have happened at any other time and I wouldn't have been there with him, but an unusual last-minute decision to change my normal evening route took me to him just as he was starting to go into sudden, acute heart failure. I crumpled to the wet ground and held him as he writhed and fought for breath, trying to work out what was happening, totally helpless to do anything for my boy except hold him and love him, like I'd held him and loved him when he was a tiny chick, just a couple of years ago. He had a traumatic, distressing death, but it was over very quickly. I don't know if it's experience or acceptance, or if one comes with the other, but even in the most traumatic circumstances, I stay quite calm, now, and hold back the shock for later. But Danny's death hit me hard. Without even a minute's warning, my pal wasn't there anymore.

I held Dan until his body started to cool, knowing it was the last time I'd feel the warmth of his life and the spark that had burned inside him and lit him up. He hadn't had the death I wanted for him, but there are a lot of decisions that aren't mine to make. I do my best and try to think of every way to keep my family safe, but there are so many things I can't control, and there's always something new to learn and change. I raked through my memory and tried as best I could to be honest with myself, but I couldn't think of anything I could have done to prevent his death, or to change how unpleasant it had been. It was what it was. He hadn't been built to last; he was born inconsequential, an unwanted by-product, doomed from the very beginning. Even in making it past a day old, Danny Carey was – literally – one in a billion, and his life wasn't inconsequential or too small to matter anymore. His life, in all its top-o'-the-cock-a-doodle-morning-to-ye, sheep-riding, camera-bag-shagging glory, mattered to him, and that's all that counted.

I couldn't sit there pondering all night; I had stuff to do. So I wiped my eyes, picked myself up and got on with the rounds.

The deaths of Bree and Danny had taken the rug out from under me. Seeing someone you love fade away is hard in ways that seeing someone you love leave so suddenly isn't, and vice versa. Their deaths had been very different, but each had taken its toll, emotionally and – in my rumbling, cramping, complaining guts – physically, too. So, although I was stubbornly bad at admitting it, Dad was right: I needed a hug.

I had some errands to do, so I took the opportunity to do them with some company. Dad and I took Baggins with us for the run, and once I'd been to the bank and post office and done some other bits and pieces, we channelled Bran and took the auld-man dog for some chips and a potter down at the park. As Baggins Hamilton careered his way round the park like it was the Castle Douglas Grand Prix, a skein of geese honked their way overhead on their journey south.

'Remember that time, up in the Cairngorms, Dad, with the geese?'

'Oh, aye – that time they got lost! That was so funny. They'd nae idea where they were going!'

It was a brilliant memory that still made us smile, decades later. Walking through the Lairig Ghru on a September weekend, many years ago, Dad and I had stood, enthralled, as a huge skein of pink-footed geese circled overhead, clearly lost, honking, *Move over, let me drive!* and *Does anybody have any idea where we are?* as they tried to navigate their way south. The funicular railway was being built on the Cairngorm mountain at the time, and we surmised that the new scar on the age-old landscape had thrown their navigation system into chaos.

'The racket they made! I think just about every one of them took a shot up front tae see if they could do any better.' I laughed. 'What a shame, though – it really threw them, didn't it?'

'Aye, they certainly weren't very happy.'

Along with spending my school holidays bottle-feeding lambs at Uncle Wull's farm and coming home from work to find seventeen kittens in my bedroom, while Mum acted like that was normal, those days spent in the hills with Dad are part of my bedrock. No matter how much I complained about my legs hurting, or having a sore head, or being hungry or cold or too tired, he always managed to encourage me to keep going (and sometimes pitted my ego against the younger kids coming up fast behind us, to motivate my malingering arse up the hill). Very rarely did my insistence that 'Daaaaaaaad, I cannae do it' win the day, and miraculously my aches and woes had usually all resolved themselves by the time we reached the cairn and the perspective-shifting views – and the Monster Munch rolls and flasks of tea – at the top. *Keep going, and if you do, there's a crisp roll in it for you* was a good lesson, learned early on.

As well as delivering a much-needed hug, Dad's *This Is Retirement?* handyman service helped me get on top of things I hadn't had time to do, which I had been lying awake worrying about instead. He restocked the food sheds, replenished straw beds and fixed and mended a few things. By the time daylight began to fade and I waved Dad off on his seventy-five-mile journey home, I'd managed to clamber back up the slippery slope a bit. I felt better after having some company and a hug. Throw in a bath, a gin and a good night's sleep, and I knew tomorrow would feel much brighter.

But before that happened, I had my nightly task of counting the chickens back into their shed.

'. . . eleven . . . twelve . . . thirteen . . .

'Awfurfuckssake, sit still! Amber, leave Joe Campbell alone. Right . . . one . . . two . . . three . . . Amber! That's plenty – *leave him alone!*'

Towards the end of the year, as the nights draw in, it often feels like, as soon as I've finished the morning rounds, getting everyone up, it's time to start the evening rounds and put everyone to bed again. I don't particularly like being out in the dark, and winter brings mud and cold – and often wind and rain and frost, too – but at least, with the birds in bed by half four and the dogs settled by seven, all else being well, winter offers the possibility of an evening to myself. Summer has its benefits, lots of them, but it's like living with 120 sleep-averse toddlers who refuse to go to bed at night. The only thing they have to do is go to bed, and they won't do it; it's the only thing I want to do, and I can't.

'Oooo, Gim, Elisa, what is it tonight, doll? Get yer snoot in there . . .'

I held the bucket for her and Gimli, while they hoovered up their lucky dip of fruit, vegetables and a few Rich Teas for good measure.

'Oh, Gim, broccoli tonight, eh? Elisa, what's that ye've got? Is that a bit of apple? Right, you pair, that's enough. Leave some for everyone else.'

I gathered up the buckets of evening snacks for the other sheep and the pigs, and nuzzled into Gimli and Elisa for a sheepy cuddle.

'Night night, you two. Night, Adam Jones. Night, Wattsicle. Night night, Flash. Love you. Sleep tight.' I gave each of the boys a kiss, and set off up the hill.

Dick had finished his own evening rounds of the farm and he was heading home for the night. Seeing my head torch bobbing its way up the hill, he tooted goodnight from the other side of the hedge on his way past; in a cold field, on a dark night, after an exhausting day, a wee friendly toot goes a long way. I've lived in a lot of places, and at Ringliggate, for the first time, I feel like I'm part of a community: friendly waves as we go about our days, passing blethers, friends' houses lit up in the dark, folk who all come at the world from different directions, who are there for each other when they need to be.

The pigs were happily demolishing cauliflowers and cabbages, and the bachelors were all settled and counted into bed. By moonlight, I headed back down the hill. It was a bright, clear night, and the grass was already starting to crunch under my feet. I went through the gate, turned to close it, and paused. The hang-oot tree at the top of the hill was silhouetted against the fading blue, and as day gave way to night, among the clouds, dots of light were starting to appear in their places. It's a nice time of day, and a lovely feeling: after a day doing what they enjoy, everyone is nestled in bed, safe, warm and content. I looked up and around at the familiar glinting spots of light, taking a few moments to think, let the dust settle, fire up the cogs and see what worked itself out.

I'd got lost in thought again, carried away on one train or other, but my hands had some sense and reminded me that it was arctic and perhaps we should think about going somewhere less cold. From behind the bushes, suddenly, a white shape emerged, waddling and bouncing at pace towards me. Every night, at bedtime, Figgy and I have a special moment together, involving a secret biscuit hidden in my pocket that only Figgy knows about.

'Meh heh heh heh!' she shouted, as she pelted towards me as fast as her dainty white legs could move her big woolly candyfloss bulk down the hill. 'Meh heh heh heh!' *Figgy knows! Figgy knows everything!* She shoved her nose through the fence and we carried out our clandestine biscuit exchange.

'Figgy knows.' I smiled as I bent down to stick my nose in her fleece for a big whiff of her slightly damp wool. 'Mwah!' I kissed the whorl of white wool on her forehead and dug my fingers into her thick fleece to give her a scratch for a few minutes while we had a chat.

'Right, darling, I'm frozen. I'm away. Night night, sweetheart. Sleep tight.' I kissed her forehead again, tucked my hands into my pockets and headed down the hill towards the warmth and the two geriatric terriers waiting to greet me in the hospice.

Badger and Digger were curled and sprawled in their respective spots in the living room, both out for the count. A few days ago, Diggity Dug had developed a huge lump on his neck. Given his age and how lumpy and bumpy he was already, I'd suspected the worst, and my heart sank as Bruce, his vet, agreed. It looked like the cancer had spread to his lymph node, and it was likely making its way around the rest of his old body. Bruce and I agreed that putting him through a whole lot of treatment was the wrong thing for him, and instead we decided to focus on making his last days as comfortable and content as they could be. I left the surgery with some antibiotics and pain relief for Digger, then we went to the supermarket and bought half the dog-treat aisle, got a bag of chips and went down the park. If he didn't have long, I was determined we were going to make every moment count. We'd only known each other for a few weeks, we'd just got into the swing of trust and friendship, and our time together was already coming to an end. *Goddammit.*

Wrapped up against the chill of a late November afternoon, the three of us walked round the park, the two auld men following their noses from one good sniff to the next, oblivious to anything but what was under their nostrils right that moment. Digs was content; if he knew he was dying, he wasn't letting it bother him. His contentment and happiness were catching, and I was so grateful to have met and fallen in love with both of them, but preparing myself for having to face saying goodbye to my new pal, just as our friendship and trust in each other was starting, was a challenge. I really felt for Badger; he knew his brother wasn't well, and it was really going to hit him hard when his best pal was gone. He'd started washing Digger's face, maybe sensing that something was wrong, and although they had their brotherly moments and I'd had to break up a few sweetie-instigated fisticuffs, they had been together their whole lives and I knew Badger was really going to miss his lifelong companion.

I'd had to hold back the thoughts to keep the tears from starting as I'd pushed the sweetie-laden trolley round Tesco, but although our time together was going to be so short, at least we'd had enough time to become good pals, and that would make everything so much easier and less stressful for Diggity Dog, and for his Badger. He could relax, enjoy his final days, and trust that the rest would be taken care of. I was really grateful to be able to give him that. It was really hard to know how to feel sometimes, but I cannae run an animal hospice and feign surprise when folk get sick and die.

A few days later, I bent down to give Digger a hug as I got him into his coat to go out for a wee. It was clear he wasn't feeling himself, and although he was eating, I was sure he'd lost weight. I was ready to listen when he told me he'd had enough, and I had a sense it wouldn't be long before I saw that look in his eyes that told me it was time to act on the promise I'd made when we'd met a few weeks ago.

'What the . . . ?' I unwrapped my arms from around him. His wee cosy jumper was soaked through, all round his neck. A wave of adrenaline washed out from my guts. Moving him into the light for a better look, I mustered my strength and focused. 'Digs, what's going on, son?' Trying to stay calm, I reassured him and lifted his head. I blinked as I took in what I was seeing: his fur was stained red, and blood was seeping out of his neck. *Shit* . . .

I called Bruce. He talked me through what to do, and within a few minutes, we'd worked out that the lump in his neck, which we'd thought was a tumour, was actually an abscess, and it had burst. As the blood and pus seeped out, the lump was getting smaller and smaller. I could hardly believe what I was seeing. I put salty water on the wound, gave him a sweetie and sat down with a cup of tea to calm myself down.

Within minutes, it was like someone had taken ten years off Digger, and a week later the lump was completely gone. He was doing pelters round the field with Badger, bouncing, and looking better than I'd ever seen him look. Much as I'm ready for death when it comes, I much prefer it when miracles pay a visit.

I tucked a blanket around Digger's back and pulled on my water-proofs. My eyes were hot and heavy. As much as I love how I spend my days, a fair amount of stress, not much sleep, no days off and responsibility that weighs me down as much as it lifts me up can make it all feel a bit fatiguing and relentless at times. I still had a few hours of stuff to do in the house, and the whole thing to do again tomorrow, but for today, everyone was settled and tucked in for the night, and it was time for lights out.

'Everybody got everything?' I had a quick check around the hospice to make sure everything was done, and ran through my mental checklist, in case I'd missed anything. *All good.* I locked the door of the hospice and stepped out into the night. 'Sleep tight, everyone. Love you.'

Gripping the day's laundry under one arm, I locked the gate and paused. Quiet and still, peacefully, everyone slept. We'd all got through another day intact. I looked up at the clear sky and the patterns of lights that dotted it. *Thank you.*

'Where is she? Black Cat, you there?'

As I was locking up one evening, a few weeks ago, a black cat had walked out of the darkness and come to meet me at the gate.

She'd wrapped herself around my legs, rolled on her back and rubbed herself all over my hands. I couldn't quite believe what I was seeing as, keeping her distance, she'd followed me into the garden and round the side of the house. I thought maybe she was a farm cat and hunger had forced her to do what was needed to survive, or maybe she'd been abandoned – though if she had been, she didn't seem remotely concerned about it. I'd pinched a couple of sachets of cat food from Archie and Josh, and the black cat had eaten four dinners, rubbed herself all over me for two hours, nibbled my fingers and then disappeared back into the darkness, leaving me sitting alone on the back doorstep, wondering what had just happened. Feral farm cat or abandoned domestic cat, that's not how cats behave. *That was weird.*

I'd asked around and folk told me that they thought she'd been living in the outbuildings at the farm for about two and a half years, which meant she would have arrived around the same time I did. She slept in the bales, and occasionally folk had caught sight of her, but she didn't go near anyone – apart from having seen a few fleeting glances of her, nobody knew anything about her. Her ear was nicked and, since she'd never had kittens, I assumed she'd been neutered, but she wasn't chipped. She was beautiful – glossy, exactly the right weight, and her eyes were healthy and vibrantly green – so she clearly knew what she was doing and was very well equipped to look after herself.

I wasn't sure if she'd come back, thinking that maybe she'd been struggling to find food as it got colder and she'd just needed a good meal and a friendly face to see her back on track. The next night, I was quite surprised when I realised how desperate I was to get back to the house and see if the black cat was there. As weird an experience as it had been, I'd really enjoyed her company.

Coming round the side of the house, I stopped in my tracks. A young rat lay twitching and panting on the path. The Black Cat had come back, and this time dinner was on her.

I shoved the day's laundry in the machine and got the tumble dryer going. Just about out of energy and enthusiasm for the day, I plonked myself on the step at the back door to send Dad our '0104' text – our code for, *Don't worry, I'm safely back in the house and I'm not under a pig or impaled on a deranged goat.* My body was feeling the strain and I could hardly think for the fatigue that closed my eyes the second I stopped and sat down. That kind of tiredness makes me weepy, and I could feel the tears of frustration, worry, loneliness and a bit of self-pity start to prick my eyes. Most days, I'm completely content being the only human here among my pals of all different shapes. As much as I love them, they love me back, and I don't think it's possible to feel unloved around this lot. For the most part, I like coming into the house exactly as I left it, doing things exactly the way I want to and being free to have gin and marshmallows for dinner, unobserved and unjudged. But I do sometimes miss the company of my own kind, with all its ups and downs and pros and cons. There are nights when I'm walking round the side of the house in the dark, usually after one of the more difficult days, and I imagine going into the kitchen to the smell of a pot of soup, being welcomed with a warm smile and hug from someone who could make everything better for a while.

'There you are!'

A pair of green eyes emerged silently from the darkness.

'Hey, Black Cat, had a good day?'

She wrapped herself around my legs, purring, rubbing against my mucky waterproof trousers. I didn't know how someone so clean and perfect, and with senses that outshone mine in every possible way, could stand the smell of me. I guess she figured that it was OK if her human was a bit rough around the edges; she'd take care of the glamour in the relationship, if I took care of the dinner arrangements.

'You ready for dinner, Black Cat?' I bowed my head to her and she rubbed her face against my forehead.

We're both naturally wary, and it's taken us a while to suss each other out, but over the weeks, the black cat and I have become very close, and the feel of her glossy black fur on my face still gives me a wee thrill. She's independent and perfectly able to look after herself, and I love her for how free and mysterious she is, but she seems to want to be with me as much as I want to be with her. Our friendship is different from the other friendships in my life. She doesn't need me. She chose me, and her decision to give me her friendship has filled up bits of me that I didn't know needed filling. I didn't know how much I needed the black cat until I met her, but thankfully *she* did. I'm glad one of us was paying attention, and I hope I can speak for both of us when I say that we are both much better off for our friendship.

Once I was sure she was going to stick around, I bought her a little house for the winter, but like any self-respecting cat, I expect she'll freely and mysteriously ignore the bloody thing.

'Come on, lassie, out for yer wee . . .'

Delighted and excited, Ri hurled herself down the stairs and out the door to empty her bladder, while I got her dinner ready. Our house is still a building site, with half-finished walls, bare floorboards, a boiler that I hope will splutter and wheeze its way through one more winter, and electrics so old and so badly wired up that I get shocks off the wall in the back bedroom, but at least there's not a pond under the dining room anymore. Ringliggate sat alone and unloved for a long time, and it still needs a lot of love and attention, but its bones are starting to heat up again and it's coming back to life. Every night, when I come into the kitchen and peel off the layers, I'm grateful for the safe, warm hug it wraps around me. There might not be a pot of soup on the stove, but there's a tray of lasagne in the fridge, waiting to be heated up for a nourishing, hot meal, and next to it, a box of brownies won't wait long to be savoured with a cup of tea at the end of a long day – nurturing care packages from Mammy Bear and my pal Lisa, reminding me how lucky I am to have people who share their kindness with me.

As well as regular calls to make sure I'm eating something that's good for me ('Brownies are good for the soul, Mum'), Mum's talent for putting thoughts and words on paper is also helping me to find the words and thoughts I need, now, to do one of the most difficult things I've ever done. Thanks to Dad's memory for details I forgot a long time ago, and my old pal Clare's obsession with books, not to mention her twenty years of knowing and understanding me, somehow, this book has come into being. Knowing how I was struggling for time, Mandy called round every day to take K-pup out for a walk, and Lisa kept all our online pals updated on daily events.

I had no idea if I could write a book, and, if I could, how I would manage to do something that seemed so unlikely and so impossible. It turns out the answer is that I spent as much time doing anything but writing as I spent doing nothing but writing, and that I wrote it falling asleep at my laptop at two a.m., I wrote it after dragging myself out of bed at five a.m., in my head while I was doing the rounds, sitting on the kitchen floor, drinking gin and eating marshmallows, and I wrote it on bits of paper ripped off a bag of oats, with a blunt Boggle pencil I found in the food shed, using a fence post as a table. But, most of all, I wrote it by remembering a lesson I learned many years ago from watching my old friend Pam: use all of yourself, all of the time, and, when you need to, use a little bit more.

The most recent panic – an emergency that means that, between us, the fencers, Craig and Gary and I are going to have to find a way to get ninety-four birds under cover in just ten days – has yet again pulled so many people together to raise the money needed to get started on making that happen. I can pick up poo, fill food dishes, give cuddles and nurse through the night, but I can't do all this alone. Without the practical, emotional and financial kindness given so abundantly and freely over the years from friends and strangers, there would be no hospice – just as, without the help and support from my mum and dad, and friends like Clare, Mandy and Lisa, I doubt I'd ever have been able to get this book finished.

When Maggie died, it seemed impossible that I'd find my way out of the labyrinth of longing, loss, love, guilt, regret and fear. I've faltered, failed, succeeded, wobbled, slid down the slippery slope and sometimes needed a helping hand back up again. Some-times, not being able to open a packet of Hobnobs was the final straw for the day/week/month/year, and I may have temporarily relinquished control of the situation to the part of me who thinks that launching a packet of Hobnobs into a pond and then having to ask a fish for forgiveness would help the situation. I've made good decisions and bad ones, but the best decision was always to keep going. Enjoy the view, follow the waymarkers along the path and, on the harder days, remember that there might be a crisp roll waiting for you at the top.

Whatever this life is, in all its wonder and horror and mystery, I know that I don't get to make the rules. I can tinker with them sometimes, but life happens, and death happens – they just do. It's part of the deal, and there's a good chance I'll never know why. I don't know far more than I'll ever know, and whatever life is, whatever death is, despite many futile attempts, I've never found a way to avoid either of them. I've figured out that things are most peaceful and easy to bear when I accept that life is going to happen, and that, at the end of it, death is going to happen, too.

If the only thing I can do is make the life bit happy, secure and full of the things that make it worth living, and make the death bit as peaceful and dignified as it can be . . . deal. I'll take it.

Over the years, so many friends have flowed into my life and ebbed out of it again, taking pieces of me with them and leaving pieces of themselves behind to fill in the cracks. Every time, it hurts like hell, and it's always too soon to say goodbye. Holding each of them as they left life behind and took the path I couldn't follow, I've learned that, whatever size and shape we come in, whatever vessel carries us through this weird and wonderful ride, when it really comes to it, in life and in death, we all want the same things.

EPILOGUE

30 December 2020

The frost was settling, and the grass crunched under my wellies as I made my way down the hill and back towards the hospice. Parts of the sanctuary that I only usually see in sunlight were lit in the moon's brilliant white glow, the same world with different highlights. I swung my hands and braced against the bitter cold finding its way through the cracks in my layers.

I stopped at the gate and looked over to the pile of freshly disturbed earth, dark and uneven against the glistening white grass. A few hours earlier, I'd watched a kind and thoughtful friend use his excavator to dig a grave and bury the Biggest, Woolliest Bastard of them all.

Gimli's twisted, wonky body was never going to last the distance. There was only so long a soul who longed for zoomies could tolerate being trapped in an irretrievably broken, failing body.

Yesterday, Gimli told me the last thing in the world I wanted to hear. This morning, I called Bruce, and he came an hour later and did the last thing in the world I wanted to do.

I looked over at the hospice. Almost three years on, it's still not finished. Recently, I've started to wonder what I would do if I had the chance to start over. I can see it in my mind's eye: the hospice in the centre of the field, with Bran's memorial garden spiralling out around it and paths reaching through the garden and up into the sanctuary. Maybe one day.

I glanced back to the mound of earth. The cut flesh is still white, and the tide is still being drawn out, but the wound will redden, and the wave will come. It'll come and it'll wipe me out, and my heart will fracture and ache, and it will hurt forever.

But I know, now, that I'll be OK, because there's only one thing powerful enough to make you do the thing you want to do least for the one you love most, and it's the most powerful thing of all.

Ebb and flow

We come and we go

Taking and leaving pieces of ourselves and each other.

ACKNOWLEDGEMENTS

Writing this book has been the hardest thing I've ever done, and, if it hadn't been for these people, there is absolutely no chance it would exist. I could never and would never have done this on my own.

Heather Bishop, who emailed me and asked me if I was interested in writing a book almost two years ago, and here we are, eighteen minutes from the deadline, and I'm still not finished. And yet, somehow, she's still not lost patience with me. Thank you for cheering me on, coaxing me into good decisions and out of bad ones, helping me through my wobbles – and always managing to find a nice way to tell me to get my arse in gear and hurry up, and to STOP BLOODY TINKERING.

Rowan Lawton, my literary agent, who has lived up to her promise of being my 'professional hand-holder' and has talked me down off the 'Why does anyone think I can write a book? I can't write a book!' ledge many times, and had faith in me when I had none.

I don't know much about the publishing industry, but surely Jane Sturrock and Charlotte Fry must be two of the most patient and understanding publishers and editors to have put up with what I've asked them to put up with. I missed every deadline, and still they trusted that one day I'd actually stop tinkering and finish the book. I finally did, and I really hope it's worth the wait . . . and the second wait . . . and the next . . .

Dad, who has put up with more than any being should have to put up with as I've cycled through every emotion and taken them all out on him. He's forgiven me for more than I can even remember, and he gave up his days to care for my family while I wrung every last word out. I really, really couldn't have done it without you, Dad. 'Whit bloody retirement?' Let's go on some walks now, eh?

Mum. Chapter finisher-off-er. Editor. All-nighter buddy. Lasagne-cheese maker and scone baker. And, no, I still don't know the difference between a colon and a semicolon; I don't think I ever will.

Clare, who gave me her time and energy, and whose suggestions and friendship are inextricably intertwined in almost every page of this book.

Jimmy L, for being my cheerleader, for reading and suggesting and believing it when he told me that I could do it.

To everyone here, who patiently waited for the promised day when it would be done and we'd have our time together again.

To the friend who had to leave before those promised moments together came. There's so much I would change.

And to the Wee Mental Ginger Dug. You made it at least twice as difficult, but I couldnae have done it without you.

To the folk who made the music that kept me company and kept me going during those long nights drinking gin and digging deep in a dark kitchen at 4am. Your magic kept me just-about sane.

In memory of two of my human pals who left while I was writing this book:

Craig, a man I only knew for a short time but whose help and friendship as he, Gary, Dad and I bonded over the *goddamnedfuckingarseholeofamarquee* will stay with me for a lifetime. You are missed, pal. But look . . . I finally finished the fuckin' thing! Telt ye . . .

Mandi, whose big heart and special soul nurtured so many folk who found their way to her. I was a lost soul myself in those early days in Aviemore, and Mandi nurtured and guided me through my first tentative steps as I felt for my path. Her wisdom will, I hope, do for others what it has done for me. You've taken and left a lot of pieces, wummin, I hope you know that.

I've got two minutes until my deadline (really), so I'll leave it there. I don't think Heather has any polite ways left to tell me to stop tinkering and just finish the bloody thing already.